ENHANCING HEART HEALTH
Preventing a Heart Attack

Matthew Budoff, MD, FACC

Forward by
David Heber, MD, PhD

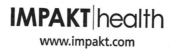

IMPAKT|health
www.impakt.com

Published by:
IMPAKT Health
2551 31ˢᵗ Street
Boulder, CO 80301
Phone: (303) 440-7402
Fax: (303) 440-7446
E-mail: info@impakt.com
www.impakt.com

ENHANCING HEART HEALTH
Preventing a Heart Attack

Matthew Budoff, MD, FACC

*"Willpower lasts about two weeks....
and is usually soluble in alcohol."*

-Mark Twain

As you read this book, remember that the ideas and suggestions put forth will not improve your health unless you maintain them. Any lifestyle modification, whether diet, exercise or product, will not help lower your cardiac risk unless you persist. This requires some time allocation and dedication on your part, but the benefit of a healthier and longer life is well worth it.

—Matthew Budoff, MD, FACC

Dedication and Acknowledgements

I would like to dedicate this book to my wife, Victoria, and son, Daniel, who put up with my long hours with a smile, and provide me the love and support I need to continue my work.

I would also like to thank those involved in the production and completion of this book:
- The executive publisher of IMPAKT Health, Karolyn A. Gazella.
- IMPAKT editors Frances E. FitzGerald and Catherine Monahan, art director Kelly Fisher, and IMPAKT publisher Miriam Weidner.
- The staff of Wakunaga of America, manufacturers of Kyolic brand garlic, especially Dr. Haru Amagase, Director, Research and Development.

—Matthew Budoff, MD, FACC

Contents

Foreword

By David Heber, MD, PhD

I began my academic career 20 years ago at Harbor-UCLA Medical Center, the institution where Dr. Budoff conducted his recent research on garlic and heart disease. Over the past 20 years, I have seen our understanding of heart disease change from a disorder largely caused by elevations in cholesterol, to a multifactorial disease caused by the interaction of our genes and the modern environment including diet and lifestyle. Obesity, which is now epidemic worldwide, has recently been associated as an independent risk factor for heart disease. In other words, obesity, independent of blood pressure, smoking, family history and gender, has a significant and detectable influence on heart disease risk.

While the connections between heart disease and obesity are not all established, obesity is clearly associated with increased levels of circulating C-reactive protein, a marker of inflammation. The cellular process of atherosclerosis is accelerated by such inflammation. Another disease associated with heart disease and obesity is type 2 diabetes. Over the next ten years, the number of individuals with type 2 diabetes is estimated to increase from 155 million to 218 million, and 80 percent of all heart disease will occur in these individuals.

Heart disease is caused by a combination of factors, a point Dr. Budoff illustrates thoroughly by discussing each of these factors directly linked to the disease. For example, while high blood pressure and high cholesterol have been linked to heart disease for decades, it was only thanks to the ground-breaking work of Dr.Kilmer McCully that the link between homocysteine and heart disease was uncovered. This discovery, coupled with modern genetic research showing homocysteine levels can be modified by an increased intake of vitamins B6, B12 and folic acid, is one of the most compelling examples of gene-nutrient interaction in human disease.

Dr. Budoff's research also provides further insights into the health benefits of garlic, which contains allyl sulfides, powerful constituents developed by the plant to fend off pests, but also of significant health benefit to humans. Thanks to Dr. Budoff's interest in cardiovascular research and his findings on garlic, his book *Enhancing Heart Health: Preventing a Heart Attack* provides a consumer friendly, easy-to-understand view into this complex topic.

Dr. Budoff utilizes current statistics and timely information to provide readers with a clear picture of the heart disease epidemic. Readers are provided with a succinct description of the workings of the cardiovascular system, as well as an overview of the multiple risk factors that can cause heart disease. The book features Dr. Budoff's innovative scientific work in diagnosis, as well as descriptions of conventional diagnostic measures and treatment techniques. As Dr. Budoff appropriately points out, if we are to change the statistics and prevent heart disease, we must follow a comprehensive plan that includes diet, lifestyle factors, supplementation and/or prescription medications. This integrative approach, which combines conventional and natural treatments, makes Dr. Budoff's plan most appealing.

Many medical doctors have been skeptical about dietary supplements. Dr. Budoff's research however, along with other studies, helps demonstrate the positive effects botanical dietary supplements can have on cardiovascular system health. Dr. Budoff's recent study involving aged garlic extract demonstrates that this natural substance can be used in conjunction with a conventionally-prescribed cholesterol-lowering medication to lower risk. Although Dr. Budoff's study was a small one, it certainly indicates the need for additional studies of this type. Almost two-thirds of all prescription drugs derive from the plant world. It makes sense to look to plant-based products such as fresh garlic and aged garlic extract supplements for health benefits for heart health.

Heart disease has certainly taken an emotional, physical, and financial toll on our society. Accurate, timely information and a clear understanding of factors that can contribute to this devastating illness are of incredible importance if we are to change the current trend. Dr. Budoff's book, *Enhancing Heart Health: Preventing a Heart Attack*, is an important addition to the current information available on heart health.

David Heber, MD, PhD, FACP, FACN is a professor of medicine and public health and the director of the UCLA Center for Human Nutrition. He is also the director of the UCLA Clinical Nutrition Research Unit, which conducts research on nutrition and cancer prevention. Furthermore, he directs the UCLA Center for Dietary Supplements Research: Botanicals and the Nutrition and Obesity Training Program. All three of these programs are funded through the National Institutes of Health.

Dr. Heber is listed in the Best Doctors in America 2002 and is listed in Who's Who in America. He has written over 100 peer-reviewed papers, two professional textbooks, and three books for the public. His research interests are nutrition and cancer prevention, obesity treatment, and botanical dietary supplements.

Introduction

Number-One Killer Disease

E very 33 seconds, someone dies of heart disease. It remains the number-one killer disease in the United States, and has held that position since 1900 (except for 1918). It is sad that symptoms and outcomes of an unhealthy heart are commonplace.

According to the American Heart Association, nearly 13 million people alive today have a history of heart attack, angina, or both. This year, more than a million Americans will suffer a new or repeat heart attack. One out of every 2.5 deaths in the United States can be attributed to heart disease. That's more than 2,600 heart disease deaths in America every single day!

The reality is that other leading causes of death pale in comparison to heart disease. Heart disease claims more lives each year than cancer, accidents, and AIDS put together. This is true in both men and women.

As a cardiologist, I am frustrated by the startling statistic that death is the first and last symptom of heart disease for almost one-third of those who have it. Of the more than 1.4 million people who died of heart disease in 2000, more than 420,000 never made it to a hospital to be treated by a physician. To a doctor who is devoted to saving lives, that fact is unacceptable.

Perhaps more disturbing is that heart disease is the number one killer of women, yet few are aware of this statistic.

Amazingly, heart disease kills more men and women each year than all forms of cancer combined. Heart disease is a blanket term that describes a category of illnesses that affect heart health. High blood pressure, cholesterol, and homocysteine levels are all thought to contribute to the development of some form of heart disease. According to the American Heart Association, of the nearly 62 million Americans with heart disease in 2000, 50 million had high blood pressure, 7.6 million suffered an acute heart attack, 6.6 million experienced chest pain or discomfort caused by reduced blood supply (also known as angina), and still another 4.7 million people suffered a stroke, a related illness caused by the loss of blood flow to the brain.

Furthermore, the American Heart Association estimates that 105 million Americans have high cholesterol, and about 42 million of those have dangerously high levels. A total blood cholesterol level of 200 mg/dl or higher is considered above normal.

The emotional and physical toll of heart disease is staggering. But the financial price we pay is also exorbitant. In 1996 alone, the American Heart Association estimated that heart disease cost the public more than $151 billion dollars. According to the most recent statistics from the American Heart Association, that number is expected to climb to almost $352 billion in 2003.

To reduce these troubling statistics and protect human health and vitality, we must first understand exactly what we are protecting and why it is so vital to do so. Let's take a closer look at the physiology of the human cardiovascular system.

Optimal Operation

When operating at peak capacity, the heart is an absolutely amazing organ. The process seems quite simple, but its

BLOOD FLOW

THE HEART IS DIVIDED INTO TWO SIDES. ONE SIDE OF THE HEART PUMPS THE "FRESH," OXYGENATED BLOOD OUT TO THE BODY, AND THE OTHER SIDE RECEIVES THE OXYGEN-DEFICIENT BLOOD.

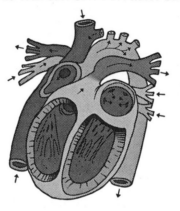

importance is monumental. After all, the result of a poorly functioning heart can be death.

The heart is a hollow muscular pump, weighing only 8 to 14 ounces, which rhythmically contracts to circulate blood throughout the body.

There are four one-way valves in the heart. As the blood is pumped, the proper valve opens to let the blood pass through. The valve then closes to keep the blood from moving backward. If the valves do not close properly, blood can leak into the previous chamber causing a reduced supply of fresh blood to the arteries. If the valves do not open efficiently, the heart has to work harder to push the blood through, which causes strain on the heart muscle.

Simply stated, the heart's main task is to move oxygen- and nutrient-rich blood out to the body's other tissues and organs, and then circulate blood from the rest of the body to the lungs where it can be reoxygenated.

After the lungs reoxygenate the blood, some is filtered through the kidneys and liver. The kidneys cleanse the blood of waste products, then eliminate the waste via urine. The liver also cleanses the blood. In addition, the liver removes and stores nutrients from the blood until they are needed. After we eat, important nutrients absorbed from the intestinal tract are dropped off into the liver via the bloodstream.

The human adult body contains anywhere from 4.5 to 6 liters of blood. Men have about 10 percent more blood than women. Amazingly, the heart pumps about 1,980 gallons of blood through our bodies every day. At rest, the heart beats about 60 to 80 times per minute. That's a lot of activity for such a small organ.

The heart is divided into two sides. One side of the heart pumps the "fresh," oxygenated blood out to the body, and the other side receives the oxygen-deficient blood. While the heart fills up with oxygen-deficient blood, it is considered "at rest." The heart contracts as it pushes the oxygenated blood out. The pressure during the resting phase is known as diastolic pressure and the pumping phase is called systolic pressure. Blood pressure readings assess both phases.

The heart methodically fills and empties, beating about 100,000 times each day. When operating optimally, this repetitive rhythm keeps us moving like a smooth-running machine. However, many factors can cause this operation to go haywire.

Something is Wrong

The seemingly simple operation of the heart is rife with risks that can damage our health or cause death. Perhaps the single, most dangerous outcome is the blockage of an artery. The arteries can become narrowed or even fully blocked as a result of plaque build up. The narrowing of an artery can occur

SYMPTOMS OF A HEART ATTACK

- Discomfort, pressure, heaviness, or pain in the chest, arm, or below the breastbone (i.e., angina).
- Discomfort radiating to the back, jaw, throat, or arm.
- A fullness, indigestion, or choking feeling (this may feel like heartburn).
- Sweating, nausea, vomiting, or dizziness.
- Extreme weakness, anxiety, or shortness of breath.
- Rapid or irregular heartbeats.

Symptoms typically last at least 30 minutes and are not relieved by rest or oral medications.

Some people have a "silent" myocardial infarction (heart attack). Although this can occur in any patient, it is more common among diabetics.

DON'T WAIT!

The best time to treat a heart attack is within 30 minutes from the onset of symptoms. Waiting can increase the damage to your heart and reduce your chances of survival. At the first signs of a heart attack call 911 for emergency treatment.

Source: Cleveland Clinic Heart Center

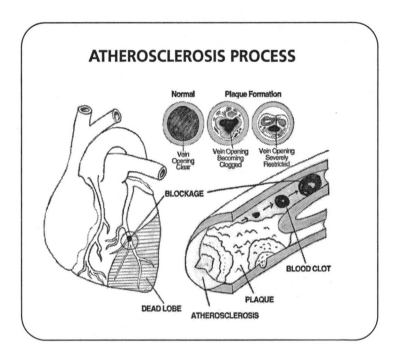

ATHEROSCLEROSIS PROCESS

anywhere in the body, but when it happens in the heart, it dramatically reduces the heart's ability to function.

It is critical that blood and oxygen move freely throughout the cardiovascular system, whether moving in or out of the heart. If this does not occur, dangerous outcomes such as those listed below may arise.

- Atherosclerosis develops when cholesterol, fat, calcification and other substances in the blood build up on the artery wall, thereby constricting the artery. This reduces the flow of oxygen-rich blood and nutrients.
- Stroke occurs when the brain sustains a sudden loss of blood flow. It is typically caused by a blood clot or a rupture of a blood vessel that leads to the brain.
- Angina pectoris is a result of an insufficient supply of oxygen-rich blood to the heart, resulting in chest pains and tightness.

- Myocardial infarction is a heart attack that occurs when the heart stops receiving blood altogether.
- Aneurysm occurs when a bulge develops in a weakened section of an artery or vein and then ruptures. It is often fatal.
- Cardiomyopathy is when the heart muscle deteriorates and becomes either enlarged, too thin, or inflexible.

Atherosclerosis is also known as "hardening of the arteries," and is one of the most common forms of heart disease in the United States. The blockage can damage the artery wall until the affected area dies. This can cause a heart attack or cardiac arrest, which happens when the heart stops beating. Even when the blockage is quite extensive, very few overt symptoms surface. All too often, the first symptom is death.

Understanding the potential results of heart disease is important, but it is even more critical to understand what causes these outcomes in the first place. We now know that multiple risk factors are involved in the development of heart disease.

PLEASE NOTE

Heart disease and its associated conditions, such as high blood pressure and high cholesterol, are serious enough to require the supervision of a qualified physician. Self-medication and/or the discontinuation of prescribed medication without the consent of your doctor can be dangerous and is not advised. If you are experiencing symptoms associated with a heart condition, seek medical care immediately.

Chapter One

Understanding Risk Factors

You can dramatically reduce your risk of being in a car accident by wearing your seat belt, driving carefully, and making sure your vehicle is running properly. These factors are all controllable. However, you can't control every factor, such as the way other people drive, the weather, or road conditions. The same is true for heart disease. You can control certain aspects that will dramatically reduce your risk of developing heart disease, but you can't control everything. In addition to identifying the factors you can and cannot control, it is important to realize that heart disease is most likely to strike when multiple risk factors are present.

The factors that you can't control include heredity (a family history of early heart disease), gender (men tend to develop heart disease earlier than women), and age (the older you are, the more likely you are to develop heart disease). People who survive the acute stage of a heart attack have a seven times higher chance of another attack than the general population.

If you have one or more of these risk factors or currently suffer from heart disease, you need to develop an even more aggressive prevention plan to help ward off heart disease.

A quick note about heredity. Just because you may have a family history of early heart disease does not mean you are destined to die of a heart attack. It simply means you have a predisposition. You can alter your destiny by using the

DO YOU HAVE HIGH BLOOD PRESSURE?

IF YOUR BLOOD PRESSURE IS HIGHER THAN 140/90, YOU ARE CONSIDERED TO HAVE HIGH BLOOD PRESSURE.

DO YOU HAVE HIGH CHOLESTEROL?

IF YOUR LDL "BAD CHOLESTEROL" IS MORE THAN 130 MG/DL OR YOUR HDL"GOOD CHOLESTEROL" IS LOWER THAN 40 MG/DL, YOU HAVE HIGH CHOLESTEROL.

prevention program outlined in this book and getting regular medical checkups.

In addition, although age is a risk factor, heart disease can begin early in life, long before you show any symptoms. This is illustrated by autopsies performed on American soldiers killed in Vietnam. Surprisingly, 45 percent of the young soldiers had some degree of atherosclerosis present in their arteries. There have been countless case histories of young individuals suddenly dying of a heart attack, even though they were not aware they had a problem. So, although age is a risk factor, it is certainly not the only factor that determines heart disease risk. Heart disease does not have to be an inevitable part of the aging process. Remember, it is caused by multiple risk factors, many of which you can control.

Controllable Risk Factors

Several conditions can increase your risk of developing a heart attack. Five of the most common are:

1. High blood pressure
2. High cholesterol levels
3. Sticky fat (LDL oxidation)
4. Diabetes
5. Elevated homocysteine

Let's take a closer look at three cardiac risk factors—elevated blood pressure, cholesterol, and homocysteine—and how they contribute to heart disease.

A blood pressure measurement is a ratio representing pressure in the arteries. The bottom number, or diastolic pressure, is the lowest pressure when the heart is relaxed. The top number, or systolic pressure, represents the highest pressure when the heart is pumping. A healthy blood pressure for adults is 120 (systolic) over 80 (diastolic).

High blood pressure, also known as hypertension, can occur when blood vessels become less elastic or arteries narrow. When diastolic pressure rises, problems can occur due to the constant strain on the arteries, even between heartbeats.

According to the National Heart, Lung, and Blood Institute (NHLBI), high blood pressure is the number-one risk factor for congestive heart failure, which results when the heart is unable to pump enough blood throughout the body.

PLEASE NOTE

NEVER DISCONTINUE A PRESCRIPTION BLOOD
PRESSURE OR CHOLESTEROL MEDICATION
WITHOUT FIRST CONSULTING YOUR PHYSICIAN.

MULTIPLE RISK FACTORS IN
CARDIOVASCULAR DISEASE

RESEARCHERS HAVE CONFIRMED IT IS A COMBINATION OF THE CONDITIONS BELOW THAT CAUSES HEART DISEASE. IDENTIFYING THE MULTIPLE RISK FACTORS, AND THEN CREATING AN APPROPRIATE PREVENTION OR TREATMENT PROGRAM TO ADDRESS THESE FACTORS, IS THE KEY TO LONG-TERM HEART HEALTH.

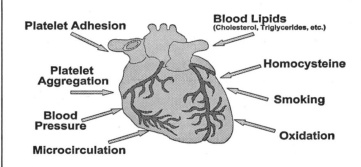

**Multiple Risk Factors in
Cardiovascular Diseases**

An estimated one-third of all strokes in the elderly are directly related to high blood pressure, particularly when the systolic number is high. High blood pressure can also damage other organs, such as the brain, eyes, and kidneys. The four main categories of high blood pressure are as follows:

1. Borderline —120 to 140 over 85 to 89
2. Mild —140 to 160 over 90 to 104
3. Moderate —160 to 180 over 105 to 114
4. Severe — 180+ over 115+

High cholesterol levels were once thought to be the single most dangerous risk factor in the development of heart disease. Although this is no longer the case, high cholesterol levels still make you more vulnerable to a heart attack.

Remember, if the blood cannot flow easily through the arteries, health problems or even death can occur. Arteries become blocked as a result of what's known as plaque buildup. This plaque is comprised of a combination of fatty material, cellular debris, calcification, and cholesterol.

But not all cholesterol is bad. The liver manufacturers cholesterol to help make sex hormones and bile acids. Without cholesterol, many body processes would be negatively affected. Also, cholesterol bound to high-density lipoproteins (known as HDL) is considered "good cholesterol" because it transports cholesterol to the liver for metabolism and elimination from the body. In contrast, cholesterol bound to low-density lipoprotein (known as LDL) is considered "bad cholesterol" because it sticks more easily to the arterial wall and builds up as plaque. That's why it is so important to know both your HDL and LDL cholesterol numbers.

The good news is that for every one percent reduction in blood cholesterol, there is an estimated two percent reduction in heart disease. To lower your risk of developing heart disease,

HOMOCYSTEINE

- WHAT IS HOMOCYSTEINE?
- WHAT IS THE RELATIONSHIP BETWEEN HOMOCYSTEINE AND CARDIOVASCULAR DISEASE?
- WHAT ARE THE BENEFITS OF LOWERING HOMOCYSTEINE?

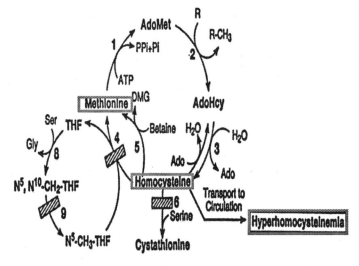

Folate in Health and Disease ed. by LB Bailey, Marcel Decker, Inc., New York, 1996.

your total cholesterol should be less than 200 mg/dl. Your LDL should be less than 130 mg/dl and your HDL should be greater than 40 mg/dl.

Homocysteine also has a powerful effect on the heart. The link between elevated homocysteine levels and heart disease has only recently been confirmed. Homocysteine is a non-essential amino acid that results from a deficiency of three B vitamins—vitamin B6, B12, and folic acid. In addition, too much dietary protein and too little of the B vitamins may help convert methionine (an essential amino acid) into homocysteine (the toxic by-product). The combination of homocysteine and LDL cholesterol contributes to plaque buildup and artery wall damage. Groundbreaking researcher Kilmer McCully, MD explains it this way: "Investigators have shown that LDL by itself is not damaging. But when it is taken up into the artery wall, it becomes oxidized or modified, and it has damaging effects on cells in the artery wall. The recent finding with homocysteine may explain why the LDL is taken up and becomes damaging to the artery wall."

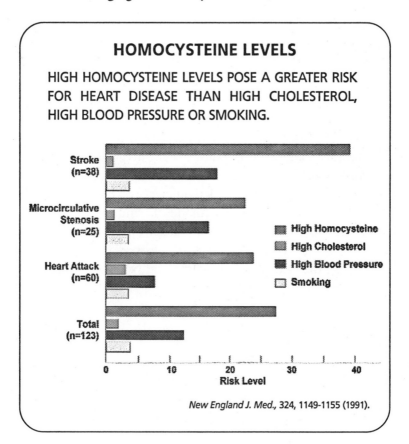

HOMOCYSTEINE LEVELS

HIGH HOMOCYSTEINE LEVELS POSE A GREATER RISK FOR HEART DISEASE THAN HIGH CHOLESTEROL, HIGH BLOOD PRESSURE OR SMOKING.

New England J. Med., 324, 1149-1155 (1991).

The research evaluating the link between homocysteine and heart disease has increased dramatically over the past few years. Recently, many of the most prestigious medical journals have confirmed the dangers of this risk factor. The *Journal of the American College of Cardiology* reported in November 2002 that elevated homocysteine levels were an independent predictor of mortality and nonfatal heart disease in patients who had undergone successful angioplasty surgery.

The February 2003 issue of *Stroke: Journal of the American Medical Association* reported that high blood levels of homocysteine significantly increased the risk of stroke in people who already have coronary heart disease. The researchers concluded: "Our findings...are consistent with a strong predictive role of [homocysteine] levels, independent of traditional risk factors or inflammatory markers, for incidence of ischemic stroke in patients at increased risk due to pre-existing coronary heart disease."

Clearly, it is important to evaluate homocysteine levels as well as cholesterol and blood pressure. Having insight about all three factors can provide valuable information about your level of risk.

How we live has a tremendous influence on the development of high blood pressure, cholesterol, and homocysteine. That means these conditions are largely within our control. If we are to reduce the rate of heart disease, we need to change the factors we can control and be aware of the ones we cannot.

The Difference Between Men and Women
One of the myths surrounding heart disease is that it is a "man's illness." However, according to the most recent statistics (Heart Disease and Stroke Statistics 2003 Update) from the American Heart Association, "...in every year since 1984,

CVD (Cardiovascular Disease) has claimed the lives of more females than males. And the gap between male and female deaths has increased dramatically..." In addition, black females are more at risk than white females. According to the statistics, a woman dies of heart disease every minute—more than half a million each year. Annually, heart disease kills 10 times more women than breast cancer.

Men and women experience and react to heart disease differently. According to the Center for the Advancement of Health, women take significantly longer to seek care for their heart symptoms than men do. Studies indicate that women usually wait more than six hours before seeking medical attention, while men wait five hours on average.

A marked difference is also apparent in the symptoms of women and men. Women typically describe their chest pain as sharp, rather than the "classic" male complaints of pressure, heaviness or tightness in the center or left side of the chest. In addition, women are more likely to describe other symptoms that are "not necessarily related to the chest pain. These symptoms include back pain, nausea, and indigestion. Thus, doctors are less likely to recognize a heart attack in women.

Improving Your Odds

High blood pressure, high cholesterol levels, and elevated homocysteine can increase your chances of developing heart disease or dying of a heart attack (refer to the sidebar on pg. 20-21). But other controllable factors can also increase your risk of these three conditions.

We will discuss the following controllable risk factors in more detail in later chapters:
• Overweight or obesity
• Lack of physical activity

THE GENDER DIFFERENCE

MEN AND WOMEN EXPERIENCE AND REACT TO HEART DISEASE DIFFERENTLY. WOMEN TYPICALLY DESCRIBE THEIR CHEST PAIN AS SHARP, RATHER THAN THE "CLASSIC" MALE PATTERN OF PRESSURE, HEAVINESS OR TIGHTNESS IN THE CENTER OR LEFT SIDE OF THE CHEST.

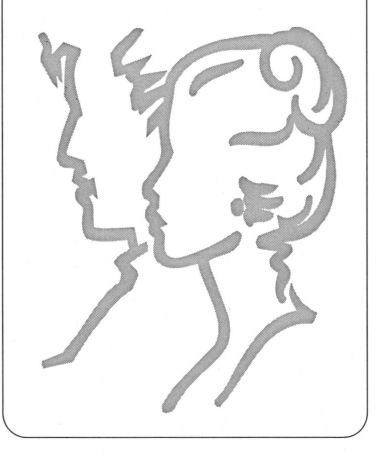

- Cigarette smoking
- Diabetes
- Increased and uncontrolled stress and anxiety
- Poor diet

Fortunately, because these factors are controllable, you can increase your odds of avoiding heart disease by making better lifestyle choices. Even more promising, if you've been diagnosed with heart disease or have had heart problems in the past, you can reverse that negative process by making positive changes. A comprehensive plan of attack is the most effective strategy.

Before we delve into the components of your comprehensive prevention or treatment plan, let's take a closer look at how conventional medicine diagnoses and treats our number-one killer disease.

Changing Risk Factors

Specific risk factors need to be addressed in order to decrease your chances of developing heart disease. The following key risk factors have been identified by the American Heart Association:

Cigarette and tobacco smoke
• Smokers' risk of heart attack is more than twice that of nonsmokers.
• Cigarette smoking is the biggest risk factor for sudden cardiac death: smokers have two to four times the risk of nonsmokers.
• Smokers who have a heart attack are more likely to die and die suddenly (within an hour) than are nonsmokers.

High blood cholesterol levels
• The risk of coronary heart disease rises as blood cholesterol levels increase.

High blood pressure
• High blood pressure increases the heart's workload, causing the heart to enlarge and weaken over time.

Physical inactivity
• Regular, moderate-to-vigorous exercise plays a significant role in preventing heart and blood vessel disease.
• Exercise can help control blood cholesterol, diabetes and obesity as well as help to lower blood pressure in some people.

- Exercise is one of the best ways of raising HDL, or "good" cholesterol.

Obesity and overweight
- People who have excess body fat are more likely to develop heart disease and stroke even if they have no other risk factors.
- Being overweight is directly linked to coronary heart disease because it influences blood pressure, blood cholesterol and triglyceride levels, and increases the risk of diabetes.

Diabetes mellitus
- Diabetes seriously increases the risk of developing cardiovascular disease.
- More than 80 percent of diabetics die of some form of heart or blood vessel disease.

In addition to these risk factors identified by the American Heart Association, new research indicates that elevated levels of homocysteine in the blood can also lead to heart disease.

High blood homocysteine levels
- Excess homocysteine can produce free radicals and oxidize cholesterol, causing damage to arteries.
- Reducing homocysteine levels requires vitamins B6, B12 and folate.

Chapter Two

Diagnosis and Treatment

I mentioned previously that 30 percent of heart attack deaths strike people who have never been properly diagnosed or treated. This makes it imperative to find better ways to diagnose and treat the disease early in its process. Individuals in that dangerous 30 percent group are what we call "asymptomatic." They continue with their daily activities, completely unaware of the dangers lurking in their cardiovascular system. Early detection is critical. It can lead the way in developing a prevention program that includes supervised lifestyle changes, further or more frequent testing, or other medical therapies.

Today, conventional medicine uses specific diagnostic techniques, prescription drugs, and surgery to help alleviate heart disease and its associated illnesses. Obviously, conventional medicine has saved many lives. However, since heart disease remains our number-one killer of men and women in all industrial nations, there is room for improvement.

Diagnosis

If we are to improve the odds, we must diagnose heart disease and its associated risk factors early. Fortunately, there are tests available that make early diagnosis possible. Blood tests determine your cholesterol and homocysteine levels. Chances are, you've had your blood pressure checked at the doctor's office on numerous occasions. The American Heart Association estimates that one in four Americans has high blood pressure. Unfortunately, nearly 30 percent of those afflicted don't even know they have hypertension. What's worse, there is no easily identifiable culprit in about 95 percent of all blood pressure cases. In other words, we just aren't sure what causes high blood pressure.

High blood pressure is often called "the silent killer" because it can develop without your knowledge. By the time it is discovered, it may be too late. That's why it is a good idea to have your blood pressure checked frequently.

Blood pressure machines are present in drugstores and hospitals. However, don't rely solely on those machines because they sometimes malfunction.

Nearly one-half of the U.S. adult population has borderline high or higher total blood cholesterol levels. It is best to check cholesterol blood levels after you have fasted for 12 hours, to ensure the food you just ate doesn't distort the reading. Your doctor will inform you of the guidelines prior to checking your cholesterol levels.

How is general cardiac health evaluated? One method used to detect blockages is the exercise treadmill test. This test causes an increased demand on the heart, and if blood supply is limited, chest pain or tightening will develop. This test can detect blockages of 50 percent or more. Any obstruction less than 50 percent will not restrict blood flow enough to produce angina or changes on the electrocardiogram. However, these mild blockages can rupture and cause heart attacks, even with a normal treadmill test. Thus, treadmill testing is not recommended for the "asymptomatic" or healthy population, as it only detects heart disease in an advanced stage.

Even more expensive tests, such as thallium tests, still can't detect obstructions that are less than 50 percent. Tragically, most heart attacks occur from lesions that create only 10 to 20 percent blockage. Even these minor blockages can rupture, causing complete blockage and possibly a heart attack.

Computed Tomography (CT) equipment has been used to detect early heart disease, but relies on a mechanical rotation of x-ray tubes, takes too long to image, and can produce blurry images of the heart. These "multi-slice" scanners also expose patients to high radiation doses. Still other tests use contrast dyes or injections to look at blood flow. However, heart disease has to be advanced before blood flow is reduced to dangerous levels.

As director of Cardiac CT at Harbor-UCLA Medical Center, I have been fortunate to be involved in a revolutionary approach to heart disease diagnosis. Electron Beam Computed Tomography (EBCT) is a convenient and quick way to get a more accurate picture of the heart. This cardiac imaging approach is seven times faster than conventional CT equipment, and can yield a full set of images very quickly. With this new technology, we can obtain scans of the heart in 1/10 to 1/20 of a second. This makes it a perfect tool to evaluate cardiac and pulmonary anatomy, blood flow, and function. These fast pictures allow for motion-free images of your heart for the most accurate assessment of heart and lung abnormalities.

NEW TECHNIQUE

ELECTRON BEAM COMPUTED TOMOGRAPHY IS A CARDIAC IMAGING APPROACH SEVEN TIMES FASTER THAN CONVENTIONAL EQUIPMENT, WHICH DIAGNOSES HEART DISEASE EARLIER THAN ANY OTHER NON-INVASIVE TEST.

It was our goal at UCLA to discover a way to make the cardiovascular diagnosis process not only simpler and more convenient for the patient, but also more accurate. EBCT allows us to do that. With EBCT, we do not evaluate blood flow. Instead, we explore the anatomy of the heart to look for any early lesions or plaque buildup before they can disrupt blood flow to the heart. Early detection allows for much earlier treatment of the plaque building up in the arteries.

The EBCT test has now been demonstrated to be a better predictor of risk than "conventional" risk factors, such as the presence of high blood pressure and high cholesterol, because it detects plaque at a very early stage. A positive scan demonstrates that plaque is building up, and the higher the "score," the greater the problem. The score is literally a volume of plaque that exists in the artery. It is estimated that persons build up detectable calcified plaque up to 10 years before the treadmill test or angiogram shows a significant problem. Thus, not only does this heart scan inform us that a person may have early plaque building, but this test gives us a number to follow over time.

In addition to physical testing, both the existing diagnosis and the EBCT program use a risk factor questionnaire. Because so many controllable lifestyle factors can contribute to heart disease, the risk factor questionnaire proves an invaluable tool in the diagnostic process.

Presently, the National Institutes of Health is studying the EBCT, and it is not widely available. I hope that, following the testing outcomes, this screening device will be used much more widely throughout the world to increase early detection and decrease dangerous disease outcomes. You can find an EBCT scanner nearest you at www.imatron.com.

Cholesterol and Blood Pressure Treatments
The medical community agrees that mild-to-moderate

cases of both high cholesterol and high blood pressure should be treated first with dietary modifications. Simple changes in diet and other lifestyle habits can usually bring mild-to-moderate high cholesterol and hypertension into the normal range. We will explore diet in the next chapter.

Some individuals with mild-to-moderate hypertension or cholesterol are put on prescription drugs. Cholesterol-lowering drugs, known as statins, make up one of the fastest growing drug categories in the United States. According to the Spring 2003 issue of the *Berkeley Science Review*, worldwide sales of these drugs have reached an amazing $30 billion annually.

Some of the more common cholesterol-lowering drugs are frequently advertised on television. This class of drugs (e.g. Pravachol, Lipitor, Mevacor, Zocor), known as statins, work by inhibiting the enzyme needed to manufacture cholesterol in the liver. However, these drugs also block the manufacture of important nutrients like CoQ10, which has been shown to benefit heart health. The other main drawback of this class of drugs is debilitating muscle pain. If you suffer from such pain consult with your physician. Other side effects, according to the *Physician's Desk Reference*, include liver problems, nausea, diarrhea, abdominal pain, headaches, and skin rash.

Despite their side effects, the statins are one of the most important methods for lowering the risk of future heart disease. These medicines have been shown to lower the chance of heart attack, stroke and death by at least one third in appropriate patients. Patients with diabetes or known heart disease (including heart attacks, strokes, bypass surgery and angioplasty patients) should be on one of these medications for the rest of their life. Patients demonstrating significant calcification in their arteries per their electron beam CT scan or an angiogram, should likewise be on these therapies.

Other persons at high risk of heart disease (like those with multiple risk factors for heart disease) should also discuss with their doctor whether they should be on one of these medications. There is no single type of intervention that has more evidence behind it in all of preventive cardiology. While not for everyone, these medications provide the backbone of preventive medicine, lowering all cardiac risks dramatically.

Are conventional treatments for high blood pressure as good? More than 80 percent of patients with hypertension fall in the borderline-to-moderate range and should use diet and lifestyle changes as a first line of treatment.

Several clinical studies, including the Australian and Medical Research Council Trials and the Multiple Risk Factor Intervention Trial, have demonstrated that high blood pressure drugs (primarily diuretics and beta blockers) offer some protection against heart disease in borderline-to-moderate hypertension.

Here is a quick look at common blood pressure medications and their side effects:

• ACE inhibitors, which are fairly well-tolerated, relax the arterial wall and reduce fluid volume. This increases blood and oxygen flow to the heart, liver, and kidneys. The main side effects are dizziness, lightheadedness, headaches, and dry cough.

• Beta-blockers, vital in patients who have suffered heart attacks and heart failure, slow the heart rate and reduce the force of contraction. In addition, they can cause fatigue, dizziness, depression, reduced libido, and impotence.

• Calcium channel blockers decrease the rate and force of contraction, relax the arteries, and slow nerve impulses in the heart. While these drugs are fairly well-tolerated, side effects include constipation, fluid retention, dizziness, headache, and fatigue.

- Diuretics have the most proven benefit of all blood pressure medications. However, they deplete potassium and magnesium (important minerals for heart health), and increase blood sugar levels, and cholesterol levels. Other side effects include muscle weakness and cramping. Blood pressure medications are among the most widely prescribed drugs in the United States today. Annual sales are estimated to exceed $10 billion.

Heart Medications

In some cases, a physician will prescribe an anticoagulant or antiplatelet drug. These types of drugs reduce blood clotting in the arteries, veins, or heart.

Anticoagulants, also called blood thinners, cause the blood to take longer to clot. Common anticoagulants are Warfarin, *(Coumadin)*, and Heparin. You should never take aspirin, *Ginkgo biloba* or vitamin E with these medications because of the risk of hemorrhage (i.e., uncontrolled bleeding).

Other side effects of anticoagulants include:
- Headaches
- Stomach pain
- Nausea, weakness, or dizziness
- Easy bruising

Antiplatelet drugs also work to prevent dangerous blood clots. Aspirin is considered an antiplatelet medicine. An aspirin a day, whether a low dose (81mg or baby aspirin) or regular dose (325mg either every day or every other day) has been shown to reduce heart attacks by 25 percent. This regimen is now strongly recommended for patients who suffer from diabetes and heart attacks. It is also recommended for others with increased risk of heart attacks, such as older patients with high blood pressure, or patients with significant coronary calcification.

In the past, menopausal women were also prescribed

hormone replacement therapy (HRT) as a way to prevent heart disease. Menopausal women are three times more likely to develop heart disease than non-menopausal women. Unfortunately, the studies indicate that HRT actually contributes to heart disease. For more information, refer to chapter four.

Surgery

From 1979 to 2000, the number of heart operations and surgical procedures increased a whopping 397 percent! That's more than 1.3 million inpatient cardiac catheterizations, 472,000 outpatient surgical procedures, and 519,000 coronary artery bypass surgeries.

A cardiac catheterization takes place when a doctor inserts a thin plastic tube into an artery or vein in the arm or leg. From there, the tube can be advanced into the heart. This procedure can be done to glean more information about heart function, to dilate obstructed arteries, or to repair certain other types of heart disease.

A new type of non-invasive angiogram is now available. This test allows doctors to see blockages with over 90 percent accuracy without requiring tubes going into the heart. This test is performed in about 20-30 minutes, most often with the Electron Beam CT scanner. This non-invasive angiogram is not yet widely available, but because of the ease, safety and cost savings, I predict it will become commonplace over the next 3-5 years.

Angioplasty involves placing a balloon at the end of a tube, which is inserted into the heart. The balloon is used to open narrow or blocked blood vessels. A metal tube, or stent, is often used to help keep the artery open.

Coronary bypass surgery is performed to "get around" clogged arteries. This major surgery can take anywhere from four to six hours. The surgeon makes an incision in the middle of the chest and separates the breastbone for easy access to the heart. In some cases of cardiomyopathy or when the heart is permanently damaged, a heart transplant may be required. Doctors also perform surgery to repair or replace defective heart valves. Risks of this surgery can include breathing problems during or after surgery, bleeding, infection, injury to nerves during surgery, or even heart attack or stroke.

Heart surgery has saved countless lives, but it is also expensive, potentially complicated, and not without risk. It is also not fool proof. Often, arteries reclog and require more surgeries. The key to successful heart disease treatment is to prevent plaque buildup from the start. The best place to begin your heart disease prevention plan is with your diet.

Chapter Three

Dangers in Your Diet

The foods we eat and the liquids we drink can provide powerful tools to enhance our health—or to destroy us. Minimizing the dangers in your diet will help you prevent and treat many illnesses, including heart disease. The acronym SAD, for the standard American diet, is appropriate on several levels. The sheer volume of food eaten each day is sad, as are the types of foods eaten. Recent estimates show that the average American eats more than 120 pounds of sugar each year. Add to that the plethora of low-fiber, high-fat foods, and you have a recipe for self-destruction. It's no wonder that most experts, myself included, consider diet one of the most important controllable risk factors for heart disease.

It's bad enough that SAD has a direct, unhealthy effect on your heart. A poor diet can also lead to obesity, one of the leading contributing factors in heart disease. According to the National Center for Health Statistics, 61 percent of all adult Americans are considered overweight or obese. Results from the National Health and Nutrition Examination Survey (NHANES II 1976 to 1980 and NHANES 1999), indicate that the rate of overweight Americans has nearly doubled in the past 20 years.

Sadly, there are also more obese children than ever before. According to NHANES 1999-2000, 8.8 million children and adolescents ages 6 to 19 are considered overweight or obese.

The number of overweight children has more than tripled during the past 40 years.

To determine whether you or your child is medically overweight, and therefore at a higher risk of developing heart disease, refer to the body mass index (BMI) chart on the next page. If the BMI calculation indicates that you're overweight or obese, you need to make dietary changes to reduce your risk of heart disease. See your healthcare provider, a registered dietitian, or a nutritionist to get assistance with the weight-loss process.

Healthy Weight, Healthy Heart

The negative effects of obesity on heart health cannot be overstated. Even individuals falling into the "overweight" category of the body mass index are putting themselves at increased risk of heart disease.

A study featured in the *Archives of Internal Medicine* (July 2001) demonstrated that the incidence of diabetes, high blood pressure, heart disease, and stroke (in men) increased along with the degree to which both men and women were overweight. Even adults who were overweight but not obese (BMI of greater than 25 and less than 30) were still at significant risk. This study even found that people in the upper range of the normal weight category (22 to 24.9) were also at increased risk. To minimize the risk of developing serious illness, the researchers suggest a BMI between 18.5 and 21.9.

A thorough analysis of your weight requires more than a number on a scale. Regarding heart disease specifically, it is the shape of your body that matters most. Individuals who carry their weight around their mid section are at higher risk. To reduce your risk, you will need to work to reduce your waist line. A waist size of less than 40 inches for men and less than 35 inches for women lowers cardiac risk and chances of

BODY MASS INDEX

Body mass index (BMI) is a measure of body fat based on height and weight, which applies to both men and women. BMI categories are:

- Underweight = <18.5
- Normal weight = 18.5-24.9
- Overweight = 25-29.9
- Obesity = BMI of 30 or greater

To calculate your BMI, go to:
http://nhlbisupport.com/bmi/

developing diabetes. An optimal heart health weight reduction program includes making your waist smaller than your hips.

If you need to lose weight, be sure to work with your doctor. It is always best to lose weight slowly, because rapid weight loss can put stress on the heart and other organs. And if you need to lose weight, don't diet! That's right. Avoid the temptation of jumping on the next diet bandwagon. Healthy, long-lasting weight loss requires a lifestyle change that includes physical activity and dietary adjustments that you can live with for a lifetime.

Diet pills and nutritional supplements containing the herb ephedra should also be avoided. These products are particularly dangerous for individuals with high blood pressure or previously diagnosed heart problems.

High protein diets have become very popular recently. While the scientific research has been mixed and this topic is still being debated, they may be appropriate for some individuals. Work with your doctor before beginning a high protein diet or any diet that dramatically changes your current eating habits.

The keys to successful weight loss are moderation and exercise. You'll find information on exercise in the next chapter.

General Considerations

When making dietary changes, you must first address the basics such as fat, cholesterol, and sodium intake. Here are the general guidelines from the American Heart Association:

• Total fat intake should not exceed 30 percent of calories.
• Saturated fat intake should not exceed 10 percent of calories.
• Polyunsaturated fat intake should be no more than 10 percent of calories.
• Monounsaturated fat should make up the rest of the total fat intake, about 10 to 15 percent of total calories.
• Cholesterol intake should not exceed 300 mg per day.
• Sodium intake should not exceed 2,400 mg (or 2.4 grams) per day.

In addition, you can make healthful food choices to help ward off heart disease. These include the following:

• Increase fiber in your diet to help rid the body of excess fats, cholesterol, and other wastes. Whole-grain breads, sugar-free cereals, pasta, and brown rice are rich in fiber.
• Eat at least five servings of fruits and vegetables each day to ensure you are getting important heart-healthy nutrients, such as antioxidants and B vitamins. Fruits and vegetables are also rich in fiber.
• Choose skim or low-fat dairy products.

- Limit your daily meat intake to no more than seven ounces, and increase your fish intake. (Eggs, legumes, and nuts are high-protein, low-fat alternatives to red meat.)
  - Drink at least six to eight glasses of fresh water each day. This helps flush sodium and maintain the proper sodium/potassium balance. It also helps flush toxins from the body and supports the kidneys and liver.
  - Eat fresh, unprocessed and, whenever possible, organic foods to avoid preservatives, additives, and food colorings.

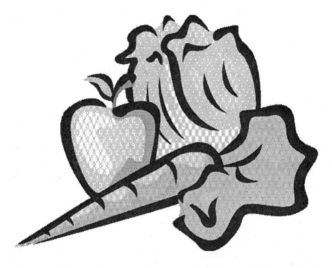

Scientific research confirms the benefits of these healthful food options. A recent study, featured in *The American Journal of Clinical Nutrition*, found that omega-3 fatty acids, like those found in wild ocean fish, can help prevent a heart attack by keeping arteries flexible. In addition to protecting against atherosclerosis, previous studies of omega-3 fatty acids demonstrated their ability to lower cholesterol and inhibit blood clot formation.

Another recent study, published in the *Journal of the American Medical Association* and in the *New England Journal of Medicine*, showed 45 percent fewer fatal heart attacks in women who ate fish five or more times per week. Finally, the April 2003 issue of *Circulation: Journal of the American Heart Association* confirmed that eating fish regularly reduced the risk of heart disease. That study revealed a 64 percent reduction in heart disease in the diabetic women who participated. This is significant because previous studies included healthy participants. Even more significant is the fact that diabetes is a risk factor in the development of heart disease.

Data from NHANES I, published in the *Archives of Internal Medicine*, indicate that eating more legumes, such as beans and peas, also reduces the risk of heart disease. Researchers conclude that legumes are especially important because they provide a wealth of soluble fiber, folic acid, and other heart-healthy B vitamins.

A study featured in the *American Journal of Clinical Nutrition* confirmed the cholesterol-lowering benefits of adding psyllium fiber to the diet. This particular study combined psyllium with the American Heart Association diet. The recommended daily intake of fiber is 25 grams. Unfortunately, NHANES III data shows that Americans only consume about 15 grams of fiber per day.

In 1999, an article in *Circulation* confirmed the health benefits of the "Mediterranean Diet." This approach emphasizes fresh fruits and vegetables, legumes, high-fiber cereals, red wine, and fish (rich in omega-3 fatty acids). The Mediterranean diet is low in cholesterol, low in saturated fat, and high in polyunsaturated fat. It appears to be an appropriate, heart-healthy option.

You may also want to add yogurt to your diet. In a recent study featured in the *European Journal of Clinical*

Nutrition, women who ate yogurt had an increase in "good" HDL cholesterol, while LDL levels remained the same. More research in this area is needed to confirm yogurt's effects on cholesterol levels.

Another interesting study featured 1,900 people previously hospitalized for a heart attack. Researchers at Beth Israel Deaconess Medical Center in Boston interviewed participants about their consumption of caffeinated tea during the year prior to their hospitalization, and then followed them for four years. The researchers discovered that, regardless of other factors (such as age, gender, and obesity), the tea drinkers tended to have lower death rates. Dr. Kenneth Mukamal, assistant professor of medicine at Harvard Medical School, reported in the *American Heart Association Journal* that the flavonoids in tea most likely provide the heart-supporting benefits. Dr. Mukamal explained that black tea, the most popular tea in North America, typically supplies the largest portion of flavonoid consumption. High consumption of coffee, on the other hand, elevates homocysteine levels in the blood.

The Anti-Inflammatory Diet

Some experts believe inflammation can lead to heart disease. Testing levels of C-reactive protein (CRP) provides healthcare professionals with a look at the body's inflammatory response. It is believed that arterial lesions containing CRP are unstable and can lead to fragments and clots.

According to Dr. Daniel J. Rader of the University of Pennsylvania School of Medicine, inflammation is "definitely a key component of plaque rupture." He adds that "Fibrinogen and homocysteine are key components in the development of clots."

One estimate indicates that individuals with high CRP levels are 4.5 times more likely to have a heart attack than those with normal CRP levels. Research indicates that reducing homocysteine levels concurrently reduces blood vessel inflammation.

A diet high in fruits and vegetables will provide B-vitamins necessary to help control inflammation and reduce homocysteine levels. Fish, olive oil, seeds and nuts are also good sources of B vitamins.

In addition to vitamins B6, B12, and folic acid, vitamins E and C have also been shown to help alleviate inflammation and contribute to overall heart health. Foods rich in vitamin E include dark green leafy vegetables. Foods high in vitamin C are citrus fruits, broccoli, red and green peppers, and spinach. Vitamin C should be taken with vitamin E because it helps regenerate oxidized vitamin E in the body.

A Quick Word About Soy

In 1999, the Food and Drug Administration began allowing food products containing soy protein to carry a label promoting soy's benefits for cardiovascular health. The labels on foods such as soy beverages, tofu, soy-based meat alternatives, and some baked goods, can now include this information if they contain at least 6.25 grams of soy protein per serving. It is believed that 25 grams of soy per day is an effective amount to benefit heart health.

Several studies have shown that soy consumption can lower cholesterol. In a 1995 meta-analysis, featured in the *New England Journal of Medicine*, researchers concluded that "consumption of soy protein, rather than animal protein, significantly decreased serum concentrations of total cholesterol, LDL cholesterol, and triglycerides, without significantly affecting HDL cholesterol concentrations."

Although more research is needed, soy consumption may also help lower blood pressure and reduce blood clotting. This makes sense because soy is a rich source of lecithin, magnesium, vitamin E, and other antioxidants shown to contribute to a healthy heart.

Blood Sugar Control

It appears that increased blood levels of insulin, a hormone produced in the pancreas, is related to weight gain and heart disease. High insulin levels can also lead to type 2 diabetes, another risk factor for heart disease. An estimated 80 percent of all adults with type 2 diabetes are obese. You can see how this all fits together.

In type 2 diabetes, the body's cells are unable to draw enough glucose (sugar) from the blood, which causes blood sugar levels to rise. The pancreas is then forced to make more insulin. As this unhealthy cycle continues, the pancreas becomes weaker and blood sugar levels are continually out of balance. Out-of-control blood sugar levels can lead to a buildup of plaque in the arteries.

Dietary diligence is the best way to avoid this problem and keep blood sugar levels in check. Follow the dietary guidelines previously mentioned, along with the following:

- Eat three meals a day. If you skip a meal, your appetite increases and your energy and blood sugar levels drop.
- If you need to snack to keep blood sugar levels balanced, choose healthy foods such as fresh fruit, carrot sticks, or unsalted nuts.
- Get to know your hunger signals so you don't overeat, and so you do eat when you are hungry.
- Remember that simple carbohydrates, such as white flour products, pasta, potatoes, corn, and bananas, can trigger greater insulin production. It's always best to choose complex carbohydrates like whole grains, vegetables, and legumes.
- Reduce or eliminate simple sugars from your diet.

Diabetes is a very complicated, serious condition. Common symptoms of diabetes include frequent urination, unusually high thirst or unexplained weight change. If you think you may have type 2 diabetes, see your doctor. If you are presently taking insulin or other medications for your diabetes, do not make any changes without consulting your physician. Type 2 diabetes is a controllable, preventable illness, and prescription medications can often be avoided. With diet and exercise, most people can stabilize blood sugar levels in a short period of time. Exercise will be discussed in more detail in the next chapter.

First Things First

To effectively prevent or treat heart disease, you must take a close look at your diet. A healthful diet has been directly linked to reduced risk of heart disease and its associated illnesses and risk factors.

JAMA reported in 2001 that drug therapy should be recommended in most cases of high cholesterol *only* after dietary modifications have been proven unsuccessful. This is also true with mild-to-moderate hypertension. However, for patients with diabetes or established heart disease, medications are often immediately recommended in conjunction with diet and exercise regimens.

Lifestyle factors are the next step. Your day-to-day choices have a colossal effect on your long-term heart health.

Chapter Four

Healthy Lifestyle—
Healthy Heart

Just as our diet has either a positive or negative effect on our health, so do our daily lifestyle choices. We decide what time to get up, what to wear, where to work, how to relax, or whom to see. Many of our choices directly and indirectly affect our heart health.

The Western scientific community is finally accepting the fact that our choices affect both our physical and emotional health. The connection between the mind and the body cannot be denied. What we think, feel, and do all have physical ramifications.

Since the turn of the 20th century, when the causes of death in the United States shifted from infectious diseases to dietary and lifestyle diseases, the effect of lifestyles on illness has been drawing more attention. In fact, in 1979, the Secretary of Health, Education, and Welfare berated Americans by stating: "We are killing ourselves by our own careless habits. You, the individual, can do more for your own health and well-being than any doctor, any hospital, any drug, any exotic medical device."

This certainly applies to heart disease. If we are to have a healthy heart, we need to practice healthy lifestyle behaviors. We may learn unhealthy lifestyle behaviors through direct, repetitive experience (something becomes a habit) or by observing the behavior of others (our parents' eating habits become our eating habits). Just as we may have learned unhealthy behaviors, we can reprogram ourselves to practice healthy behavior. It's time to create new habits.

Many studies have demonstrated that dietary intervention, along with consistent exercise, can reduce heart-disease risk factors like high cholesterol and hypertension. A study of obese participants, featured in the *European Journal of Clinical Nutrition*, showed a 17 percent reduction in cholesterol levels, an 11 percent drop in blood pressure, and a four percent decrease in weight. The participants followed an 1,800-calorie-per-day diet, received weekly counseling, and participated in moderate aerobic exercise.

Physical Activity Is The Most Important

Exercise is perhaps the most powerful medicine available. Many studies have confirmed the wide range of health benefits of consistent physical activity.

Recently, the *New England Journal of Medicine* published information from the Women's Health Initiative Observational Study, which tracked the walking, vigorous exercise, and hours spent sitting of nearly 74,000 women, ages 59 to 79. At the beginning of the study, the women had not been diagnosed with cardiovascular disease. At the end of the trial, researchers discovered that the lowest rate of heart disease events were in the women who did the most walking and vigorous exercise. The opposite was true for the women who spent more time sitting.

Other studies have shown that exercise can:
• Stimulate a positive immune response
• Release "feel-good" endorphins in the brain
• Increase oxygen and blood flow
• Increase bone density and muscle mass

For these and other reasons, exercise is not only beneficial for heart disease, it can also help with depression and anxiety, osteoporosis, fatigue, diabetes, and weight loss. In addition,

HEART RATE CALCULATION
TO CALCULATE YOUR MAXIMUM HEART RATE,
SUBTRACT YOUR AGE FROM 220. NEXT,
CALCULATE 60 TO 80 PERCENT OF THAT FIGURE.
THE RESULT IS YOUR TRAINING HEART RATE.

exercise has been shown to increase stamina, relieve pain, increase mental sharpness, improve sleep quality, and promote longevity. Exercise can keep you feeling and looking younger. No pill or surgical procedure available can do all that!

Here is how exercise directly boosts heart health and lowers the risk of heart attack:

- It reduces body fat, thereby protecting against dangerous, extra weight.
- It uses up excess sugar in the bloodstream, making cells more sensitive to insulin and reducing the chance of plaque formation.
- It has been shown to increase HDL cholesterol levels and decrease LDL cholesterol levels, thereby reducing a key risk factor.
- It conditions the heart to pump more efficiently.
- It can also lower blood pressure by dilating arteries, veins, and capillaries.

NOTE: Before beginning a new exercise program, consult a physician, especially if you have a history of heart disease or high blood pressure.

There are three key components to any effective exercise program:

1. Aerobic activity
2. Stretching
3. Strength training

Aerobic activities, such as running, swimming, brisk walking, and cycling, should bring the heart rate up to 60 to 80 percent of your maximum rate for 30 minutes. In addition to reducing the risk of injury or strain, stretching increases blood flow, improves flexibility, and prepares the body for exercise. You can do some simple stretches before and after your workout. Asian movement exercises, such as yoga, tai chi, and qi gong can also effectively loosen tight muscles and improve strength, flexibility, and coordination.

Strength training increases bone density and muscle mass while building strength. By increasing lean muscle, strength training speeds up your metabolic rate so you can burn more fat. A strength-training program may involve free weights, resistance machines, resistance bands, or water resistance in a pool. You may want to get the help of an experienced trainer before starting a program. The benefits of strength training make it worth the extra effort. You will feel stronger and more energetic than ever before.

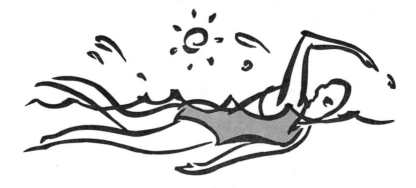

Here are some important exercise guidelines to consider:
- Make exercise or some type of physical activity part of your daily routine.
- The best exercise program incorporates at least 30 minutes of aerobic activity at your training heart rate (see calculation sidebar) for a minimum of four days per week. Keep in mind that if you have not exercised in a while and have been fairly inactive, you may not be able to exercise at this pace in the beginning. But stay focused; you will be surprised how quickly you get into shape.
- It is better to exercise at the lower end of your training heart rate for a longer period of time than at a higher intensity for a shorter period of time. It is also best to exercise four times a week for 30 minutes than two times a week for one hour.
- Choose activities that you enjoy and be sure to mix them up. Make exercise fun. That way you are more inclined to keep doing it.
- Wear comfortable clothing and shoes that fit correctly.
- Write down your goals and tell a friend or family member what they are. People tend to stick with an activity if they have goals and are accountable to them.
- Once you get into better shape, enhance your program by setting new goals and stepping up the pace.
- You may find that an "exercise buddy" will help you stick with a program and make your exercise routine more enjoyable.
- Don't forget the warm-up and cooldown phases. A warm-up can protect against muscle injury. A proper cooldown gradually returns your body to its normal state, which is important for your cardiovascular system. The cooldown phase, which is often overlooked, can include walking and should taper off in intensity.

You look and feel better when you're in shape. Exercise can help prevent and even reverse heart disease. It is one of the most important, healthy lifestyle activities you can choose.

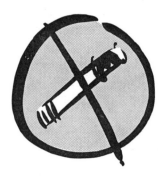

Don't Smoke!

Cigarette smoking is the single, most dangerous lifestyle activity you can choose. No credible scientific or medical organization would dispute the link between smoking and heart disease. Smoking causes heart disease and can trigger a heart attack.

According to the American Heart Association, cigarette smoking has declined since 1965. However, based on 2002 statistics, nearly 50 million American adults still smoke. Almost 26 percent of the male adult population and 21 percent of women smoke, clearly putting themselves and those around them at risk of premature death due to heart disease or cancer.

It is not easy to quit smoking. However, the benefits of quitting are almost immediate. The World Health Organization has reported that just one year after quitting, a previous smoker's risk of heart disease decreases by 50 percent. Within 15 years, the risk of dying from heart disease for an ex-smoker is almost identical to a person who has never smoked. Your heart will reap the benefits of the effort you make to quit smoking.

TIME TO QUIT

Quitting smoking may be the most difficult thing you do and it may also be the most important. It's not easy to quit smoking, especially if you have been smoking for a long time. Fortunately, countless individuals have proven that it is possible. The "stop smoking success stories" have utilized one or more of the following techniques to kick their habit:

• **Acupuncture**—Although there have not been clinical studies on the effectiveness of acupuncture to help an individual stop smoking, there are plenty of testimonials. It appears that acupuncture can help people cope with the intense symptoms of withdrawal.

• **Cold Turkey**—The withdrawal symptoms are more intense when you simply stop smoking without any assistance; but if you can make it through the first two weeks, you have a great chance of succeeding.

• **Exercise**—Not only is exercise healthy for the heart, it can also be a great way to channel energy and release endorphins ("feel-good" chemicals in the brain). Exercise is a positive activity you can use to replace smoking.

• **Hypnotherapy**—This technique is used to alter the subconscious mind to help alleviate your dependence on smoking. There are no clinical studies that confirm hypnotherapy's effectiveness, but many people have benefited from this technique. ➤

TIME TO QUIT cont.

• **Props**—Gum chewing, holding a cigarette without lighting it, and eating celery or carrot sticks, are a few activities that can help keep you from smoking.

• **Support**—Keeping a journal may help release tension caused by smoking withdrawal. Also, be sure to surround yourself with family and friends who are supportive of your decision to quit. Focus on the positive reasons for quitting, like saving money and enhancing your health. Recognize your smoking triggers and avoid them or replace them with positive activities.

• **Prescriptions**—Nicotine replacement therapy can help smokers get used to not smoking gradually. Drugs such as Zyban actually give the brain a nicotine buzz without the cigarette. Unfortunately, there are side effects with these drugs. Gum and nasal spray are also available. Be sure to discuss options with your doctor.

The best approach to quitting is a comprehensive one that includes as many techniques as possible to remain smoke-free. If you fail, try again. It's worth the extra effort and your heart will reward you by helping you be more vital and healthy than ever before.

If you find it difficult to quit smoking for yourself, do it for those around you. Children, for example, are dramatically and negatively affected by second-hand smoke. Children exposed to second-hand smoke have a higher incidence of asthma and allergies, and are much more likely to smoke as teens and later as adults.

A study recently presented at the American College of Cardiology in Chicago further demonstrates the negative effects of second-hand smoke. Researchers evaluated admissions at St. Peter's Community Hospital in Montana, where a smoke-free ordinance went into effect in June 2002 and was suspended in a legal challenge six months later. Researchers at St. Peter's discovered that the number of heart-attack victims fell by nearly 60 percent in that six-month period. This study is the first to show that smoke-free environments directly help prevent heart attacks. Other studies have shown that second-hand smoke affects cardiovascular function within minutes of exposure.

Smoking causes heart disease on a number of different levels:

1. Inhaled carbon monoxide reduces oxygen flow.
2. Increased adrenaline speeds up heart rate, constricts arteries, and raises blood pressure.
3. Chemicals in tobacco smoke damage blood vessels, stiffen artery walls, and contribute to plaque formation.
4. Oxidation occurs, increasing blood clotting and inflaming arteries.
5. Smoking also increases LDL and lowers HDL cholesterol.

New research from Tulane University indicates that smokers have higher blood levels of three clotting and inflammation factors: C-reactive protein, fibrinogen, and homocysteine. All three have been linked to heart disease.

According to Dr. Daniel J. Rader, Director of Preventive Cardiology at the University of Pennsylvania School of Medicine, this study "suggests that the impact of smoking is not so much on plaque buildup itself but on factors that promote plaque rupture." This explains why the risk of heart attack drops significantly soon after a person stops smoking.

The American Heart Association's position is that "cigarette smoking is the most important and preventable cause of premature death in the United States."

Double Check Your Meds

Physicians prescribe medications for your health. Paradoxically, blood pressure and other medications may, in fact, cause heart problems.

JAMA recently made national headlines when it reported that the newer, aggressively advertised COX-2 inhibitors (Vioxx and Celebrex) for arthritis increase the risk of heart attack. Doctors sometimes prefer these anti-inflammatory medications because they don't cause peptic ulcers, as do non-steroidal anti-inflammatory drugs (NSAIDs), such as ibuprofen and naproxen. Based on this new study, many physicians are rethinking their position.

Researchers at the Cleveland Clinic conducted the study, which featured about 16,000 patients. In the study, patients taking the COX-2 inhibitor were more than twice as likely to suffer a cardiovascular event such as heart attack, angina, or stroke.

If you are presently taking a COX-2 inhibitor or hormone replacement therapy, and are concerned about the risks, talk to your doctor about other options. Also talk to your doctor if you are taking other medications and are not sure about their effect on your heart. It is always prudent to understand how different medications may interact and what potential side effects may occur.

In addition, specific medications deplete the body of important heart-healthy nutrients. Here are some examples:

- Diuretics deplete magnesium, potassium, zinc, and CoQ10.
- Aspirin and NSAIDs deplete folic acid.
- Corticosteroids deplete calcium, vitamin D, potassium, zinc, vitamin C, magnesium, folic acid, and selenium.
- Oral contraceptives deplete folic acid, vitamins B6, B2, and B12, vitamin C, magnesium, and zinc.
- Estrogen products deplete B6, magnesium, and zinc.
- Some antidepressants deplete B2 and CoQ10.
- Some antacids deplete calcium, folic acid, and B12.

If you take any of these medications, talk to your physician about using dietary supplements.

The Latest on Hormone Replacement Therapy

Menopausal women have been told for decades that if they take hormone replacement therapy (HRT), they will reduce their risk of developing heart disease. The most commonly prescribed HRT includes a combination of estrogen and progestin (Prempro).

Scientific studies have indicated that estrogen increases "good" cholesterol and decreases "bad" cholesterol. It has then been assumed that estrogen, when taken in drug form, will reduce the risk of developing heart disease. Numerous studies, including the recently widely publicized Women's Health Initiative (WHI) have shown that HRT does just the opposite: it actually increases a woman's risk of developing heart disease.

The WHI was originally planned as an 8.5 year study to assess the risk to benefit of Prempro. The potential dangers to the study participants were viewed to be so significant that the study was halted after five years. The WHI included more than 16,000 women. Results demonstrated that women had a much higher risk of developing coronary heart disease

(CHD), stroke, and venous thromboembolism (a clot in the cardiovascular system). The researchers concluded: "Overall health risks exceeded the benefits from use of combined estrogen plus progestin for an average of 5.2 year follow-up among healthy postmenopausal US women. The risk-benefit profile found in this trial is not consistent with the requirements for a viable intervention for primary prevention of chronic disease, and the results indicate that this regimen should not be initiated or continued for primary prevention of CHD."

For menopausal women, utilizing the program outlined in this book will provide a much safer way to prevent heart disease compared to using HRT. Unfortunately, many women still suffer from menopausal symptoms that HRT can help alleviate. These symptoms include:

• Hot flashes and/or night sweats
• Insomnia
• Anxiety and/or depression
• Poor concentration and/or memory problems
• Fatigue
• Urinary incontinence
• Reduced libido and/or vaginal dryness

For women experiencing these symptoms, I suggest trying a natural approach that includes a dietary supplement or supplements. Adding soy to the diet has helped some women combat menopausal symptoms. In addition, some herbs containing phytoestrogens can naturally mimic estrogen activity without the side effects.

If you are a menopausal woman and interested in preventing heart disease, discuss HRT alternatives with your doctor. Your local natural health store will have an herbal supplement(s) containing the phytoestrogens mentioned above.

Control Stress

When you think about stress, you may imagine difficult deadlines at work, overwhelming financial pressures, crying children at home, or the illness of a loved one.

We all face world stressors, economic stressors, family stressors, work stressors, and relationship stressors. How do we cope with all this stress?

To protect your heart and overall health, you need to make a valiant effort to control your reactions to stressors. Many studies have confirmed the link between long periods of high stress and heart disease. Here's why.

Your body physically reacts to perceived stressors with what is called the fight-or-flight response. This response is hard-wired into the human system. It pumps out extra adrenaline so you can either attack or flee from danger. Unfortunately, you react to stress this way even when you face no immediate physical danger. When the "fight-or-flight" mode lasts too long or occurs too frequently, it can damage your health.

Think about the last time you were stressed out. Did your palms sweat, did your heart race, did your breathing become more shallow? That was your body moving into action, and it thought it was doing you a favor. Your body can't tell the difference between the stress of a tight deadline, the death of a loved one, or the threat of fire. As long as you view the situation (no matter what it is) as stressful, your body goes into overdrive.

Famous stress researcher Hans Selye cites the three stages your body goes through (refer to chart on the next page):

1. Stage of Alarm
2. Stage of resistance
3. Stage of exhaustion

During the alarm stage, powerful hormones such as cortisol, epinephrine, and norepinephrine are released. When the body remains on this high-alert level for an extended period, adrenal burnout occurs.

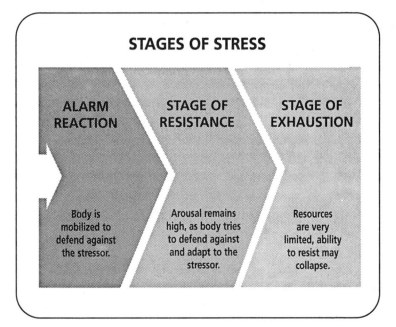

STAGES OF STRESS

ALARM REACTION

Body is mobilized to defend against the stressor.

STAGE OF RESISTANCE

Arousal remains high, as body tries to defend against and adapt to the stressor.

STAGE OF EXHAUSTION

Resources are very limited, ability to resist may collapse.

During the stage of resistance, the body tries to adapt to the stress. The alert phase is diminished somewhat, but the body remains at attention. It tries to replenish the hormones released during this stage, but its ability to cope with new stressors has weakened. According to Selye, we are most vulnerable during this stage to what he called "diseases of adaptation." Heart disease and associated conditions, such as hypertension and high cholesterol levels, can develop during this phase.

During the exhaustion phase, the body loses its ability to fight back. If the stress continues, illness is sure to develop.

According to the widely used Social Readjustment Rating Scale, the top 25 stressors are, in order:

1. Death of a spouse
2. Divorce
3. Marital separation
4. Jail term

5. Death of a close family member
6. Personal injury or illness
7. Marriage
8. Fired at work
9. Marital reconciliation
10. Retirement
11. Change in the health of a family member
12. Pregnancy
13. Sexual difficulties
14. Gaining a new family member
15. Business readjustment
16. Change in financial state
17. Death of a close friend
18. Change to a different line of work
19. Change in the number of arguments with spouse
20. A mortgage more than $10,000
21. Foreclosure of mortgage or loan
22. Change in responsibilities at work
23. Son or daughter leaving home
24. In-law troubles
25. Outstanding personal achievement

You can see from this partial list that even positive events, such as retirement, marriage, pregnancy, and personal achievement, can be considered stressful. While this rating scale is not definitive, it does illustrate the variety of life events that many people view as stressful.

Naturally, there are stressors you can control and stressors you cannot control. While you cannot control job layoffs, for example, you can control your reaction to the stressor. You can take positive steps to find a new job, such as updating your resume and networking. You can also take good care of your body and mind so you can better cope with stress.

The following ideas may help you deal with and reduce your stress load:

- Exercise is a great stress reducer.
- Meditation has been shown to relax the mind and calm the body.
- Aromatherapy oils (e.g., lavender) and some herbal teas (e.g., chamomile and valerian) have a calming effect.
- Massage and other body work can help you unwind.
- Listening to relaxing music, reading a good book, or taking a hot bath might be the perfect way to end your day.
- Taking a relaxing walk during your lunch hour or after dinner may help you relieve work tensions.
- Journaling your thoughts and feelings can help you release anger, fear, and frustration. Once the thoughts are written down, it is easier to let them go.
- Seeing a therapist or counselor during exceptionally stressful times may be helpful.
- Talking to friends or family members about your stress may also be necessary.

Caution: It is often tempting to participate in unhealthy behaviors during times of elevated stress. Those behaviors only cause more stress. So, avoid the following negative activities when trying to reduce your stress:

- Do not drink alcohol or use recreational drugs to relieve stress.
- Do not overeat or eat unhealthy foods.
- Do not rely on prescription or over-the-counter drugs unless you are under the supervision of a healthcare professional.
- Reduce or eliminate caffeine from your diet. Caffeine puts additional stress on your adrenal glands.
- Avoid extreme behavior. Too much work, too much sleep, too much of anything can be damaging.
- Do not isolate yourself.

Stress reduction expert, Leslie Reisner, Ph.D., sums up stress in this way, "Not all stress is bad. In fact, all of us need some stress in our lives to challenge and motivate us. However, prolonged, unmanaged stress can have negative physical and mental health consequences. Long term stress can cause headaches, ulcers, skin irritations and can significantly increase your chances of developing heart disease, high blood pressure, diabetes or immune system problems. In addition, experiencing high levels of stress for long periods of time can cause you to lose sleep, feel fatigued, angry, depressed and have trouble concentrating. Prolonged stress can also lead to harmful "coping" behaviors such as procrastination and using substances to relieve stress. Since it is unrealistic and undesirable to eliminate all the stress in your life, one must learn how to manage stress more effectively. Healthy stress management includes learning how to change dysfunctional behaviors, challenging unproductive thoughts and improving relaxation practices. Stress is part of being alive, the goal is to handle it more effectively."

You need to manage stress in healthy ways so your body can rebound and rebuild. If you can't create stress-free zones in your life, you will increase your risk of heart disease and heart attack.

Deal With Depression

Besides stress, depression can also damage the heart. Furthermore, depression and stress can be a dangerous combination. However, depression alone can effectively erode health.

Statistics from the National Institute of Mental Health for 2001 indicate that about 11 million Americans suffer from chronic mild depression during the course of a year.

How do you know if you are experiencing clinical depression versus the common, occasional blues? According to the American Psychiatric Association's Diagnostic and Statistical Manual of Mental Disorders, if you have at least four of the following symptoms nearly every day for at least two weeks, you are probably clinically depressed:

- Poor appetite and significant weight loss, or increase in appetite and significant weight gain.
- Insomnia or increased sleep.
- Agitation or sluggishness in movement and thought.
- Loss of interest or pleasure in usual activities.
- Decreased sex drive.
- Fatigue and loss of energy.
- Feelings of worthlessness, self-reproach, or excessive or inappropriate guilt.
- Diminished ability to concentrate, or indecisiveness.
- Recurrent thoughts of death, suicide, or suicide attempts.

Several studies have identified a direct link between depression and an increased risk of developing heart disease. For example, a study published in the *Archives of Internal Medicine* reported that elderly people with high blood pressure have more than twice the risk of developing heart failure if they are also depressed.

Following the heart-healthy dietary recommendations outlined previously will also help relieve depression. In addition, specific nutritional supplements and lifestyle factors can lift your mood. Not surprisingly, consistent exercise has proven to be an effective, nontoxic antidepressant. A recent study in the *British Journal of Psychiatry* reported that older, depressed adults reduced their depression rating by 30 percent following participation in a 10-week exercise program.

Clinical depression is a serious condition and requires medical supervision. If you feel you are clinically depressed, see your doctor. If you are presently taking antidepressant medication, do not discontinue it without first consulting your physician.

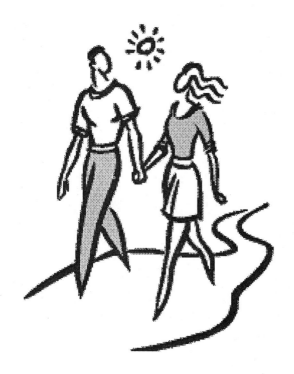

Love and Support

In his book *Love & Survival: The Scientific Basis for the Healing Power of Intimacy*, Dr. Dean Ornish writes, "When you feel loved, nurtured, cared for, supported and intimate, you are much more likely to be happier and healthier. You have a much lower risk of getting sick and, if you do, a much greater chance of surviving."

Several scientific studies confirm Dr. Ornish's conclusions, especially regarding heart health. This shouldn't surprise us; after all, isn't the heart the organ of love? Here are a few examples of the more interesting studies on love and health:

- Researchers at Yale focused on 119 men and 40 women who had angiographies. Those who felt the most loved and supported were found to have substantially less blockage in their arteries than other participants.
- A study in Sweden found that women who felt they had deep, emotional relationships also had less coronary artery blockage.
- Researchers from Case Western Reserve University found that of the 10,000 married men they studied, those who felt loved by their wives had significantly less chest pain, even though they had other risk factors.
- The "Beta-Blocker Heart Attack Trial" investigated more than 2,300 men who had survived a heart attack. Researchers found that the men classified as being socially isolated, with a high level of stress, were four times more likely to die than the men who were not considered socially isolated and had lower stress levels.

The health-damaging effects of loneliness and isolation are well-documented. So are the health-enhancing effects of love and support.

To enhance the health of your heart, keep these three simple rules in mind:

1. Surround yourself with loving, supportive people.
2. Give as much love and support as you need to receive.
3. Love yourself.

Ornish writes, "...love promotes survival. Both nurturing and being nurtured are life-affirming."

Chapter Five

Supplementing For Best Results

Even with the most meticulous diet and consistent exercise routine, some individuals may require a little more "insurance" to help keep their heart pumping strong. Dietary supplements contain vitamins, minerals, herbs, and other nutrients to fortify the diet. These are available over-the-counter without a prescription.

Here are some key reasons you may benefit from dietary supplementation.

- Overprocessing of foods has depleted important nutrients.
- The preservatives, additives, hormones, and artificial flavors and colors, contained in nonorganic foods rob your system of important nutrients.
- Smoking, alcohol abuse, and other negative lifestyle factors deplete nutrients.
- Illnesses such as depression, diabetes, and high blood pressure can weaken body systems.
- Some individuals may need additional nutrients. For example, menopausal women may need more calcium and magnesium than they can easily obtain from their diets, and older men may require additional zinc.

Chances are, if you have had heart problems or a family history of heart disease, you probably need dietary supplements, too.

Unfortunately, many dietary supplements are available, and much conflicting information is published, that your buying decision can be more complicated than necessary. Although this book is not intended to be the definitive guide to heart-healthy dietary supplements, it is important to review a few of the more scientifically substantiated nutrients and herbs. One of the most widely studied supplements for heart health is aged garlic extract. We will discuss garlic and the new study I have just completed in greater detail. But first, let's take a look at a few other compounds you may want to try.

Consider These Nutrients

Earlier we touched on the dangers of high homocysteine levels. In addition to aged garlic extract, vitamins B6, B12, and folic acid can help keep homocysteine levels in check. The formulation of these three nutrients and aged garlic extract has been shown to lower homocysteine levels. Wakunaga of America holds an exclusive U.S. patent on this formulation.

A study featured in the *New England Journal of Medicine* confirmed B6, B12, and folic acid help keep arteries free of plaque. In this study, patients who had undergone successful angioplasty were given either placebo or the B vitamins. After six months, the group receiving the B vitamin combination had only half as much renarrowing of the arteries as the people who took a placebo. The researchers concluded: "This inexpensive treatment, which has minimal side effects, should be considered as adjunctive therapy for patients undergoing coronary angioplasty."

The Swiss heart study featured in the *Journal of the American Medical Association* evaluated the ability of these three vitamins to lower homocysteine levels. More than 550 patients were evaluated. The study demonstrated that "homocysteine-lowering therapy with folic acid, vitamin B12, and vitamin B6 significantly decreases the incidence of major adverse events" in patients with established heart disease. In addition to vitamins B6, B12, and folic acid, fish oils have demonstrated impressive benefits for heart health. As I mentioned in the dietary section, fish has been linked to improved heart function. Fresh fish contains important essential fatty acids (EFAs). Unfortunately, many Americans either don't like fish or are just not eating enough of it. For this reason, fish oil supplements are available.

My Most Recent Study

I was involved in a year-long research study at the Research & Education Institute (REI) at Harbor-UCLA Medical Center. This randomized, double-blind, placebo-controlled study followed 19 cardiac patients. Nine of the patients were given an aged garlic extract supplement while the other 10 were given placebo. At the end of the study, the patients taking the aged garlic extract had significantly less coronary plaque formation than those in the placebo group. The aged garlic extract group also had lower blood homocysteine levels. (The study used Kyolic brand aged garlic extract.)

All the patients in this study were also taking cholesterol-lowering drugs. The patients who took the aged garlic extract showed a tendency toward reduced LDL and increased HDL cholesterol levels. Our study demonstrated that aged garlic extract not only prevented plaque buildup, it also positively affected two significant risk factors for health disease—high cholesterol and elevated homocysteine.

Even though this is a small study, my team and I are very excited about the findings. Our research suggests that aged garlic extract may significantly benefit people with existing cardiovascular risk factors, or those who already have heart disease. This could have a radical effect on the health of our nation and the quality of life for high-risk individuals.

Why did we choose aged garlic extract? It is perhaps one of the most widely studied natural substances for heart health presently available. More than 350 scientific studies completed at major universities have included aged garlic extract. These studies have focused on garlic's effects on:

- Cholesterol
- Blood pressure
- Homocysteine levels
- The stickiness of LDL cholesterol
- Blood thickness
- Blood circulation

While other natural substances and most prescription drugs work on one risk factor (cholesterol, for example), the scientific evidence confirms that aged garlic extract can help prevent and reverse multiple risk factors. Because heart disease is rarely caused by just one risk factor, this is especially significant.

Strong Research on a Powerful Substance

As a research scientist, I am delighted to see that the medical literature features such positive, strong research on aged garlic extract. My research has demonstrated the multiple benefits this substance has on heart health. The chart on the following page shows just some of the important research done on this powerful natural substance.

Garlic promotes heart health by acting in many different ways:

- Anticlotting
- Antiplaque
- Reducing high LDL cholesterol and raising HDL cholesterol levels
- Lowering blood pressure
- Antioxidant activity
- Lowering homocysteine levels

CARDIOPROTECTIVE EFFECTS OF GARLIC FOUND IN VARIOUS CLINICAL STUDIES

	IMPROVEMENT%
PLATELET ADHESION[1,15] (sticking together)	35-58
PLATELET AGGREGATION[1,15] (clumping/clotting)	10-25
LDL CHOLESTEROL[2, 3, 6, 7]	5-12
TOTAL SERUM CHOLESTEROL[3, 4, 6, 7]	6-31+
TRIGLYCERIDES[4, 5, 6]	10-19
BLOOD PRESSURE[3, 6]	6-8
HOMOCYSTEINE[8, 9]	24-35
LDL OXIDATION[10, 16] (sticky bad cholesterol)	35-51
SMOKING CAUSED OXIDATIVE DAMAGE[11]	29-48
MICROCIRCULATION[12, 13, 14]	67

1. Steiner, et al., J. Amer Coll. Nutr., 13(5):524, 1994
2. Yeh, et al., J. Amer Coll. Nutr., 13(5):545, 1995
3. Steiner, et al., Amer J. Clin. Nutr., 64-866-870, 1996
4. Lau, et al., Nur Res.,7:139, 1987
5. Kawashima, et al., Shinryou To Shinyaku (Treat. New Med.) 26:377-388, 1989
6. Steiner, et al., Shinryou To Rinsho (New Drug Clin.) 45(3):456-466, 1996
7. Yeh, et al., In Food Factors for Cancer Prev., 226-230, 1997
8. Amagase, H. Method and Pharm. comp for reducing serum cy conc. US Patent # 6, 129, 918, 2000
9. Yeh, et al., FASEB J. 13(4):A232; # 209.12, 1999
10. Munday, et al., Atherosclerosis, 143:399-404, 1999
11. Rahman, et al., J Nutri., 132:168-171, 2002
12. Kikuchi, et al., Jpn. J. New Remedies Clin., 43(1):146-158, 1994
13. Okuhara, T., Jpn. Pharmacol. Therapeut. 22(8):3695-3701, 1994
14. Yokoyama, K, et al., Oyo Yakuri (Appl. Pharmacol), 36:301-308, 1998
15. Steiner and Li, J. Nutr., 131:980S-984S, 2001
16. Lau, et al., J. Nutr., 131:985S988S, 2001

You'll find a complete listing of references on aged garlic extract at the back of the book. Feel free to take this book and show the references to your physician. They will assure you and your doctor about the scientific nature of the information provided.

When combined with a healthy diet, exercise, and appropriate lifestyle choices, aged garlic extract can dramatically reduce your risk of developing heart disease and possibly help you prevent another attack.

The Best Form of Garlic

While you may have previously thought of garlic as simply a great way to make foods more flavorful, it is actually a very complex herb. The chemical makeup of garlic is quite intricate. In addition to sulfur compounds, garlic contains many valuable nutrients, including calcium, magnesium, potassium, vitamin C, and selenium.

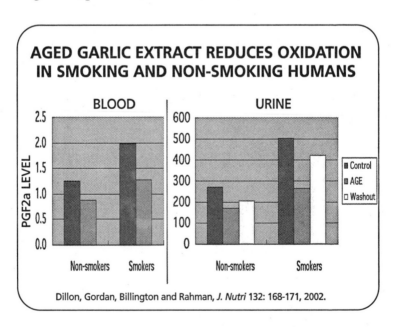

AGED GARLIC EXTRACT REDUCES OXIDATION IN SMOKING AND NON-SMOKING HUMANS

Dillon, Gordan, Billington and Rahman, *J. Nutri* 132: 168-171, 2002.

SCIENTIFIC DOCUMENTATION

MORE THAN 350 SCIENTIFIC STUDIES CONDUCTED
AT MAJOR UNIVERSITIES HAVE BEEN COMPLETED
ON AGED GARLIC EXTRACT.

Raw, fresh garlic may cause stomach upset. It is also very sensitive and reactive. If you crush or heat garlic, for example, the chemical constitution of garlic changes. Heating garlic actually destroys many of its health-promoting components.

Slowly aging garlic without heat creates a product that is concentrated, valuable, stable, and safe. The aging process also increases the amount of S-allyl cysteine (SAC) in the garlic. SAC is a water-soluble, sulfur-containing antioxidant that has been directly linked to improved heart health. It is also known to protect the liver.

One unique aging process, which can last up to 20 months, converts unstable, harsh, and highly pungent components of fresh garlic into more beneficial, less odorous compounds. The odorous compounds are not responsible for garlic's beneficial effects, and decreased odor makes people much more likely to comply with dosage recommendations. The garlic used in aged garlic extract should be grown organically so it is free of pesticides and herbicides. Only the aging process truly takes care of garlic odor in the most safe and effective manner. Many garlic products claim to be odorless, but only mask the odor with chemicals or sugar coatings. When these capsules or tablets dissolve in the body, garlic odor can result.

Two other forms of garlic, presently on the market in tablet or capsule form, are garlic oil and garlic powder. Both use heat or some other harsh processing method that destroys many of the active compounds in garlic. Fresh garlic, which is typically used in cooking is also available. However, we now know that crushing and/or heating also changes the makeup of garlic. Comparative studies have demonstrated aged garlic extract's superiority over fresh garlic and other garlic products for heart health, liver health, and immune system function. Some garlic manufacturers standardize their products based on their allicin content. However, further study indicates that allicin is highly unstable and breaks down very easily. In a report published in the *American Journal of Nutrition*, researchers concluded, "...allicin is only a transient constituent of garlic preparations and does not pass through the intestines or enter the bloodstream. No allicin is absorbed from the gut into the liver. Injected allicin is rapidly destroyed in the blood." It is unlikely that allicin is the reason garlic is so effective.

New Research on How It Works

Recently, researchers at Pennsylvania State University discovered one of garlic's most important mechanisms of action. Dr. Yu-Yan Yeh and his colleagues found that SAC, the important ingredient in aged garlic extract helps inhibit the liver's ability to produce cholesterol. This significant finding demonstrates that aged garlic extract works similarly to cholesterol-lowering drugs but without the side effects.

Dr. Yeh concludes, "Aged garlic extract can be useful for the general public to help achieve the desired cholesterol level of 200 or less." Dr. Yeh also states that aged garlic extract can be used in conjunction with cholesterol-lowering drugs. This confirms our recent findings, and is still another reason why I recommend consumers use aged garlic extract versus other forms of garlic.

Aged garlic extract is available as a dietary supplement at most natural health stores and pharmacies throughout the world. Just be sure to ask for aged garlic extract.

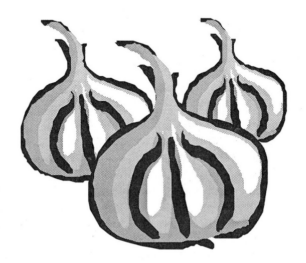

Garlic's Safety Record

As a physician, I need to know how safe a substance is. Doctors are directed to "First, do no harm." I take that direction very seriously. So it is important to pay close attention to drug interactions (sometimes called contraindications), toxicity, and side effects.

Garlic's great safety record is another reason why I chose to use it in my study. Several preclinical and clinical toxicity tests have established the safety of aged garlic extract.

Raw garlic, on the other hand, has some alarming side effects when taken in excess. Raw garlic can cause anemia, bleeding ulcers, depression, weight gain, and reduction in red blood cell count. It can also cause diarrhea and dehydration, low blood sugar, and decreased sperm levels. Most of the side effects of raw garlic are linked to the oil-soluble constituents and are not present in aged garlic extract.

MY PLAN AT A GLANCE

To review, the following are important guidelines that can help you prevent a first or repeat heart attack, or treat an existing heart condition:

1. Work with a qualified healthcare professional. Consult your physician about using aspirin, blood pressure and cholesterol medications.
2. Identify your risk factors.
3. Make diet and lifestyle changes to reduce or eliminate controllable risk factors.
4. Take aged garlic extract each day to help keep the cardiologist away.
5. Identify other appropriate supplementation.

Recommended dietary guidelines include the following:
- Reduce sodium and saturated fat intake.
- Increase daily fiber consumption.
- Eat a minimum of five servings of fruits and vegetables daily.
- Eat more fish and less red meat.
- Drink plenty of fresh water each day.
- Eat organic foods whenever possible.
- Add soy to your daily diet.

Lifestyle factors to keep in mind include:
- Daily physical activity.
- Relaxation to control stress levels.
- Smoking cessation.
- Weight control through diet and exercise.
- Loving and supportive people in your life.
- Treatment of related illnesses, such as depression and diabetes.

The aging process substantially reduces the toxicity of raw garlic. Even when large doses are taken, aged garlic extract is nontoxic. This has been shown in acute and subacute toxicity tests, chronic toxicity tests, mutagenicity tests (concerning mutation and changes in the cells), and general toxicity tests. Clinical studies involving more than 1,000 participants have also reported no serious side effects from the long-term consumption of aged garlic.

Garlic may increase the action of blood-thinning medications such as *Warfarin* (Coumadin). If you are taking a prescription anticoagulant, consult your physician before taking garlic. Also, tell your physician if you are taking garlic before you undergo any type of surgery.

Work With Your Doctor

If you are concerned about preventing a heart attack, whether you have previously had heart problems or not, you should work closely with your doctor. Although many cardiologists or general practitioners are not necessarily inclined to utilize a more natural approach, it is still critical to talk openly with your doctor about your desire to do so.

Be sure to inform your doctor about everything you are presently taking, including nutritional supplements. And remember, you have the right to make your final decision. Your doctor is your resource. You are the decision-maker. Utilize your doctor's expertise fully and then make your decision based on what's best for you in your individual circumstance.

It Takes a Comprehensive Approach

As you can tell, I am impressed with the cardiovascular-protective and treatment potential of aged garlic extract.

However, I would never recommend that you simply take a garlic pill and ignore all the other factors that contribute to heart disease. We must use all the tools we have if we are to prevent and treat heart disease. The most effective approach is a comprehensive one. The bad news is that heart disease continues to have a stranglehold on Western society. The good news is that you can make a dramatic difference to benefit your heart. In large part, heart disease is preventable, and existing heart problems can be reversed. With a comprehensive plan that covers diet, lifestyle, and dietary supplements such as aged garlic extract, you can increase your odds of avoiding a heart attack and living a long and vital life.

Appendix

Heart Terms and Definitions

Angina

A sudden intense pain in the chest, often accompanied by feelings of suffocation, caused by a momentary lack of adequate blood supply to the heart muscle.

Anticoagulant

An agent that prevents or retards coagulation, especially of the blood.

Antiplatelet

An agent which interferes with the ability of platelets (small particles of cells in the blood which promote clotting) to aggregate and form a platelet plug. It is a mild form of blood thinning.

Aorta

The main vessel in the arterial network, which conveys oxygen-rich blood from the heart to all parts of the body, except the lungs.

Artery

A tubular, thick walled muscular vessel that conveys oxygenated blood from the heart to various parts of the body.

Atherosclerosis

A type of "hardening of the arteries" in which cholesterol, fat and other substances in the blood build up in artery walls. The arteries to the heart may become narrowed, cutting down the flow of oxygen-rich blood and nutrients to the heart.

Blood Pressure

The pressure of the blood against artery walls. It is recorded in millimeters of mercury as two numbers: the systolic (maximum pressure as the heart contracts) over the diastolic (minimum pressure when the heart is at rest).

Calcification

A part of the atherosclerosis process, which is readily detected and measured by Electron Beam Computed Technology.

Cardiomyopathy

A disease of the heart muscle that can result in muscle enlargement, lack of flexibility, or a thinning of the heart muscle tissue.

Cardiovascular diseases

Conditions that affect the heart and blood vessels, including heart disease and stroke.

Cholesterol
A soft, waxy substance produced by the body and found in food of animal origin. It is needed for functions such as making hormones. Blood cholesterol is the amount of cholesterol circulating in the bloodstream.

Congestive heart failure
A condition that occurs when the heart loses its ability to pump blood. The term suggests that the heart stops suddenly and completely. However, heart failure usually develops slowly and symptoms may not appear for years.

Coronary
Refers to the blood vessels that supply blood directly the heart and is often used to refer to the heart and to heart disease.

Diabetes
A disorder characterized by the inadequate production or utilization of insulin, which is a hormone essential for proper metabolism of blood sugar.

Heart disease
A condition that affects the heart and its arteries. It includes such conditions as coronary heart disease, valve disorders, arrhythmias, cardiomyopathy (a disease of the heart muscle), congestive heart failure and endocarditis (an inflammation of the lining of the heart and its valves).

Homocysteine

A non-essential amino acid that can become toxic if it is not converted to methionine, an essential non-toxic amino acid.

Hypertension

The medical term for high blood pressure. Hypertension can often be controlled or prevented.

Lipids

Lipids are fatty substances such as cholesterol and triglycerides located in blood and body tissues.

Risk Factors

Habits, traits or conditions that increase a person's chance of developing coronary heart disease. There are two types: those that can be modified and those that can't. Modifiable risk factors include: cigarette smoking, high blood pressure, high blood cholesterol, being overweight, physical inactivity, and diabetes. Uncontrollable risk factors include gender (men tend to develop heart disease earlier than women), heredity (family history of early heart disease) and age (45 and older for men; 55 and older for women).

Statins

A category of commonly prescribed cholesterol-lowering drugs.

Stroke

A sudden loss of function of part of the brain due to loss of blood flow. It may be caused by a clot (thrombosis) or rupture (hemorrhage) of a blood vessel to the brain.

Triglycerides

Lipids carried through the bloodstream to tissues. They are obtained mostly from fat in foods. Most of the body's fat tissue is in the form of triglycerides, which is stored for use as energy.

Valve

A structure that allows blood to flow through the heart in one direction only.

Veins

Any tubular vessels that carry oxygen-depleted blood to the heart.

Ventricle

A small chamber of the heart that fills with blood and then contracts to move the blood to the arteries. There are two ventricles in the heart.

References

1. UCLA study, *FASEB J.* 2003, April 15, 2003, San Diego.
2. Lau, B., Lam, F. *et al.* 1987. *Nutr. Res.* 7:139-149.
3. Silagy, C., Neil, A. 1994. *J. Royal Coll. Physic.* Lond. 28(1): 39-45.
4. Warshafsky, S., Kamer, R. *et al.* 1993. *Ann. Intern. Med.* 119: 599-605.
5. Kawashima, Y., Ochiai, Y., *et al.* 1989. *Shinryou To Shinyaku (Treat. New Med.)* 26: 377-388.
6. Yeh, Y., Lin, R. *et al.* 1995. *J. Am. Coll. Nutr.* 13:545.
7. Yeh, Y., Lin, R. *et al.* 1997. In Food Factors for Cancer Prevention. Ohigashi, *et al.* eds., p 226-230. Springer-Verlag, Tokyo.
8. Steiner, M., Lin, R. *et al.* 1996a. Shinyaku To Rinsho *(New Drug Clin.)* 45(3): 456-466.
9. Steiner, M., Lin, R. 1994. *J. Amer. Coll. Nutr* 13(5): 524.
10. Steiner, M., Lin, R. *et al.* 1996b. *Am. J. Clin. Nutr.* 64: 866-870.
11. Rahman K., Billington, D. 2000. *J. Nutr.* 130: 2662-2665.K.
12. Rahman K. *et al.*, 3rd International Congress on Phytomedicine (3rd ICP), Munich (Germany) October 11-13, 2000.
13. Steiner, M., Lin, R. 1998a. *J. Cardiovascular Pharmacol.* 31: 904-908.
14. Steiner, M. 1998b. Recent Advances on the Nutritional Benefits Accompanying the Use of Garlic as a Supplement. Newport Beach, CA. November 15-17, 1998b.
15. Steiner, M., W. Li, *J. Nutr*, 131: 980S-984S (2001).
16. Steiner, M. *et al.*, 3rd International Congress on Phytomedicine (3rd ICP),Munich (Germany) October 11-13, 2000.
17. Yokoyama, K, Fuwa, T. *et al.* 1988. *Oyo Yakuri Appl. Pharmacol.* 36: 301-308.
18. Kikuchi, N., Nishimura, Y., *et al.* 1994. Shinyaku To Rinsho Jpn. *J. New Remedies Clin.* 43(1): 146-158.
19. Okuhara, T. 1994. *Jpn. Pharmacol. Therapeut.* 22(8): 3695-3701.
20. Steiner, M., Lin, R. *et al.* 1996b. *Am. J. Clin. Nutr.* 64: 866-870.
21. Ohnishi, S.T., Ohnishi, T. *et al.* 2000. *Nutrition* 16: 330-338.
22. Takasu, J.MD, PhD, *et al.* BMC Blood Disorders, June 2002, 2:3.
23. Ohnishi, S.T. Therapeutic Use of Specially Processed Garlic for Sickle Cell Disease. US Patent # 6,254,871; July 3, 2001.
24. Khalid, Q., Sultana, L. *et al.* 1994. Pak. J. Sci. Ind. Res. 37(12): 524-527.
25. Qureshi, A., Lin, R. *et al.* 1990a. First World Congress on the Health Significance of Garlic and Garlic Constituent, Washington, D.C. August 28-30, p. 16.
26. Abuirmeileh, N, Lin, R. *et al.* 1991. FASEB J. 5: A1756.
27. Yu, S., Qureshi, N. *et al.* 1991. National Conference on Cholesterol and high blood pressure. Sponsored by Cholesterol Education Program of the National Institutes of Health. April 8-10, 1991, Washington, D.C.

28. Liu, L. and Yeh, Y.Y. 1998. *FASEB J.* 12(4): A261 #1523.
29. Liu, L. and Yeh, Y. 1999. *FASEB J.* 13(4): A556; #442.7.
30. Yeh, Y. 1999. Recent Advances on the Nutritional Benefits Accompanying the Use of Garlic as a Supplement. Newport Beach, CA. November 15-17, 1998.
31. Liu, L. and Yeh, Y. 2000. *Lipids* 35(2): 197-203.
32. Yeh, Y.Y. and L. Liu, J. *Nutr*, 131: 989S-993S (2001).
33. Liu, L. and Yeh, Y. 2001. Orange County Convention Center, Exhibit Hall A4. April 4, 2001.
34. Gupta, N. and Porter, T. 2001. *J. Nutr.* 131: 1662-1667.
35. Liu, L. and Yeh, Y. 2001. *Lipids* 36(4): 395-400.
36. Liu, L. and Yeh, Y. 2002, *J. Nutr.* 132: 1129-1134.
37. Qureshi, A., Lin, R. *Et al.* 1990. First World Congress on the Health Significance of Garlic and Garlic Constituents. Washington, D.C. August 28-30, p. 37.
38. Yeh, Y. and Yeh, S. 1994. *Lipids* 29(3): 189-193.
39. Efendy, J, Campbell, J. *et al.* 1996. *J. Vasc. Res.* 33(S1): 23.
40. Amagase, H., Moriguchi T., and Kasuga, S. 2000. *Phytomed.* 7(2): 118.
41. Moriguchi, T., Itakura, Y. *et al.* Recent Advances on the Nutritional Benefits Accompanying the Use of Garlic as a Supplement. Newport Beach, CA. November 15-17, 1998.
42. Moriguchi, T, N. Takasugi, and Y. Itakura. *J. Nutr*, 131: 1016S-1019S (2001).
43. Qureshi, N., Lin, R., *et al.* 1990b. First World Congress on the Health Significance of Garlic and Garlic Constituents. Washington, D.C. August 28-30, p. 17.
44. Yu, S., Qureshi, N., *et al.* National Conference on Cholesterol and high blood pressure. Sponsored by Cholesterol Education Program of the National Institutes of Health. April 8-10, 1991, Washington, D.C.
45. Abuirmeileh, N., Lin, R. *et al.* 1991. *The FASEB J.*, 5: A1756.
46. Yeh, Y., Yeh, S. *et al.* 1999. *FASEB J.* 13(4): A232; #209.12.
47. Amagase, H. 2000. Method and pharmaceutical composition for reducing serum homocysteine concentrations. Patent #6,129,918.
48. Lee, E., Steiner, M. *et al.* 1994. *Biochim. Biophys. Acta* 1221:73-77.
49. Efendy, J, Campbell, J. *et al.* 1997. *Atherosclerosis* 132: 37-42.
50. Efendy, J, Campbell, J. *et al.*. 1996a. *J. Vasc. Res.* 33(S1): 23.
51. Efendy, J, Campbell, J. *et al.* 1996b Proceedings of the 1996 Conference of the Anatomical Society of Australia and New Zealand, Brisbane, Australia, p. 19.
52. Campbell, J.H., Efendy, J.L. *et al.* Recent Advances on the Nutritional Benefits Accompanying the Use of Garlic as a Supplement. Newport Beach, CA. November 15-17, 1998.
53. Campbell, J.H, J.L. Efendy, N.J. Smith, and G.r. Campbell, J. *Nutr*, 131: 1006S-1009S (2001).
54. Ide, N. *et al.*, 3rd International Congress on Phytomedicine (3rd ICP), Munich (Germany) October 11-13, 2000.

55. Ohnishi, S. Recent Advances on the Nutritional Benefits Accompanying the Use of Garlic as a Supplement. Newport Beach, CA. November 15-17, 1998.
56. Ohnishi, S.T. and T. Ohnishi, J. Nutr, 131: 1085S-1092S (2001).
57. Ohnishi, S.T., Ohnishi, T., et al. 2000. Nutrition 16: 330-338.
58. Ohnishi, S., Ohnishi, T. and Ogunmola, G. 2001. Blood Cells, Molecules Dis. 27(1): 148-157.
59. Slowing, K., Ganado, P. et al. Recent Advances on the Nutritional Benefits Accompanying the Use of Garlic as a Supplement. Newport Beach, CA November 15-17, 1998.
60. Slowing, K et al., J. Nutr, 131: 994S-999S, 2001.
61. Matsuura, H. Recent Advances on the Nutritional Benefits Accompanying the Use of Garlic as a Supplement. Newport Beach, CA. November 15-17, 1998.
62. Matsuura, H. Cholesterol lowering effects of saponins from garlic. 2000. Phytomed. 7(2): 48.
63. Matsuura, H et al.: Cholesterol lowering effects of saponins from garlic, 3rd International Congress on Phytomedicine (3rd ICP), Munich (Germany) October 11-13, 2000.
64. Matsuura, H., J. Nutr, 131: 1000S-1005S, 2001.
65. Amagase, H. et al. 2000. Ch. 6. Phytochemicals and Phytopharmaceuticals. AOCS Press, Champaign, Illinois, pp. 62-78.
66. Garlic Fluidextract. United States Pharmacopeia-National Formulary (USP25 NF20). United States Pharmacopeial Convention. Rockville, MD, p. 2553, 2002.
67. Abuirmeileh, N., Yu, S. et al. 1991. FASEB J, 5(6):A1756, #8048.
68. Munday, J. et al. 1999. Atherosclerosis 143: 399-404.
69. Ide, N. and Lau, B.H.S. 1997a. FASEB J. 11(3): A122/#713.
70. Ide, N., Lau B.H.S. et al. 1997a. Planta Med. 63: 263-264.
71. Ide, N. and Lau, B.H.S. Recent Advances on the Nutritional Benefits Accompanying the Use of Garlic as a Supplement. Newport Beach, CA. November 15-17, 1998.
72. Ide, I and. Lau, B.H.S J. Nutr., 131: 1020S-1026S, 2001.
73. Lau, B.H.S. Recent Advances on the Nutritional Benefits Accompanying the Use of Garlic as a Supplement. Newport Beach, CA. November 15-17, 1998.
74. Lau, BHS, J. Nutr., 131: 985S-988S, 2001.
75. Ho, S., Ide, N., and Lau, B. 2001. Phytomedicine 8(1): 39-46.
76. Ide, N. and Lau, B. Phytomed. 6(2): 125-131, 1999.
77. Ide, N., Lau, B.H.S. 1999. Drug Dev. Industr. Pharm. 25(5): 619-624.
78. Ide, N. and Lau, B. 1997c. J. Pharm. Pharmacol. 49: 908-911.
79. Steiner, M. and Lin, R.I. 1998. J. Cardiovascular Pharmacol. 31: 904-908.
80. Morihara, N., et al. 2002, Life Sci., 71: 509-517.
81. Yamasaki, T., Lau, B. et al. 1994. Phytother. Res. 8:408-412.

82. Lin, R.I. 1990. First World Congress on the Health Significance of Garlic and Garlic Constituents. Washington, D.C. August 28-30, 1990, p. 22.

83. Center for the Advancement of Health. *Facts of Life*. March 2000, 5:3.

84. Reuters Health. *Medline Plus*. 2002.

85. Bazzono, LA., He, J., Ogden, LG., *et al*. *Arch Intern Med*. 2001; 161: 2573-8.

86. He, J., Ogden, LG., Vupputuri, S., *et al*. *JAMA* 1999; 282:2027-34.

87. Abramson, J., *Arch Intern Med*. 2001; 161:1725-1730.

88. Mukherjee D, Nissen SE, Topel EJ. Risk of Cardiovascular events associated with selective COX-2 inhibitors. *JAMA* 2001; 286(8);954-9.

89. Tice, JA., Ross, E., Coxson, PG., *et al*. *JAMA* 2001; 286:936 – 43.

90. Schnyder, G., Roffi, M., Pin, R., *et al*. *N Engl J Med* 2001; 345:1593.

91. Sartorio , A., Lafortuna, CL., Vangeli, V., *et al*. *Eu J Clin Nutr* 2001; 55:865 – 69.

92. Hu, FB., Bronner, L., Willett, WC., *et al*. *JAMA* 2002; 287:1815 – 21.

93. Albert, CM., Campos, H., Stampfer, MJ, *et al*. *N Engl J Med* 2002; 346:1113 – 8.

94. Hu, FB., Circulation: *Journal of the American Heart Association*. April 1, 2003.

95. De Lorgeril, M., *et al*. Circulation: *Journal of the American Heart Association*. February 16, 1999.

96. Walker, A. Of Hearts and Herbs. *The European Journal of Herbal Medicine*. 1997. 3: 20-24.

97. Mashour, NH., Lin, GI., Frishman, WH. *Archives of Internal Medicine*. 1998. 3: 2225-2234.

98. Anderson, JW., Davidson, MH., Blonde, L., *et al*. *Am J Clin Nutr*, 2000; 71:1433 – 8.

99. Arky RC (medical consultant). *Physician's Desk Reference*, 52nd Edition, 1998.

100. Pelton R, LaValle JB, Hawkins EB, Krinsky DL. *Drug-Induced Nutrient Depletion Handbook*, 1999-2000.

101. Hulley S, Furberg C, *et al*. *JAMA* 288(1):58-66, 2002.

102. Seethaler S: *Berkeley Science Review*, Spring 2003.

103. Field AE, Coakley EH, Must A, Spadano JL, Laird N, Dietz WH, Rimm, Colditz GA. *Arch Intern Med* 161(13):1581-1586, Jul 9, 2001.

104. Tanne D, et al. *Stroke: Journal of the American Heart Association*, Feb 21, 2003.

105. Schnyder G, Flammer Y, Roffi M, Pin R, Hess OM. *J AmColl Cardiol*, 40(10):1769-1776, Nov 20, 2002.

106. Bazzano LA, *et al*. *Annals of Internal Medicine* 138:891-899, 2003.

107. Budoff MJ, Georgiou D, *et al*. *Circulation* 1996;93:898-904.

108. Budoff MJ. Prognostic Value of Coronary Artery Calcification. *J Clin Out Manag* 2001:8;42-48

109. Collins R, Armitage J, *et al*. *Lancet*. 2003;361:2005-16.

110. Sever PS, Dahlof B, *et al*. *Lancet*. 2003;361:1149-58.

111. Budoff MJ, Lane KL, *et al*. *Am J Cardiol* 2000;86:8-11

112. *Mastering Stress 2001- A LifeStyle Approach*, David H. Barlow, Ph.D., Ronald M. Rapee, Ph.D., Leslie C. Reisner, Ph.D. American Health Publishing Company, Dallas Texas, 2001.

IMPAKT|health

www.impakt.com